RADIANT HEALTH

RADIANT HEALTH

The Ancient Wisdom of the Chinese Tonic Herbs

RON TEEGUARDEN

WARNER BOOKS

A Time Warner Company

Author's Note

The information presented in this book is derived from traditional and modern texts and from oral teachings reflecting the observations of numerous authorities on Chinese herbs. This information should not be used to diagnose, treat, or attempt to prevent any disease without the advice of a qualified physician familiar with your medical history and condition, as well as a qualified health practitioner knowledgeable about Chinese herbs. The Chinese tonic herbs are traditionally used to promote health, not counteract disease. If you are suffering from any ailment that may require medical attention, do not consume herbs unless advised to do so by a physician.

Warner Books, Inc., 1271 Avenue of the Americas,
New York, NY 10020
Visit our Web site at http://warnerbooks.com

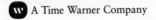 A Time Warner Company

Printed in the United States of America
First Printing: July 1998
10   9   8   7   6   5   4   3   2   1

Library of Congress Cataloging-in-Publication Data
Teeguarden, Ron.
   Radiant health : the ancient wisdom of the Chinese tonic herbs /
Ron Teeguarden.
     p. cm.
  Includes index.
  ISBN 0-446-51898-0
  1. Herbs—Therapeutic use. 2. Tonics (Medicinal preparations)
3. Medicine, Chinese. I. Title.
RM666.H33T444 1998
615'.321'0951—dc21   97-41029
                                               CIP

Acknowledgments

I wish to express my gratitude to the three great academicians who have helped me in gathering information for this book and who have taken the time, at various stages of the project, to review the material and provide me with sound advice and profound wisdom: Xu Guo-Jun, Wang Zheng-Tao, and Zhou Zhen-He. I also wish to express my gratitude to Yan Yin Pan, Yin Yun Qing, and especially to my wife, Yanlin Teeguarden, for helping me in innumerable ways in the creation of this book.

Contents

Foreword

Health is everything. Health is all. Health is the most precious treasure anyone can possess. Without health, our life would be dull—no happiness, no success, a great loss. "Health and longevity!" is the most sincere and pleasing greeting presented by Chinese people. This book, *Radiant Health*, written by Ron Teeguarden, will help you to discover a marvelous field of healthcare. Hopefully, it will help you use some of the tonics and achieve radiant health.

The art of radiant health has been widely practiced for thousands of years by the people of the East. In China, you will find that this healthcare art has permeated into almost every corner of life. Tonic teas, foods, and wine are familiar to and appreciated by all the people of the East. But Westerners may find them mysterious, inconceivable and somehow ridiculous. Now

Ron Teeguarden's book provides a powerful glass through which you in the West can easily spy on the secrets of the Chinese healthcare arts.

The classical Chinese philosophies and theories on nature and the human body may be the biggest obstacle for Westerners to learning and practicing a program for radiant health. With his profound knowledge about Chinese civilization, the author of this book has successfully kicked the big stone away and can therefore lead the readers smoothly into the great palace of Chinese radiant health. Readers will find in Chapters 1 through 3 of this book that the principles of the Chinese art of radiant health have become simple and understandable due to the author's clear and accurate interpretations and descriptions. We really appreciate it very much.

The author's brief introduction to Chinese herbalism and tonic herbs is also just to the point. Through it, readers can easily learn and grasp how Chinese tonic herbs are classified, selected, and used. All the tonics and herbal formulations listed and introduced in this book are the classical ones or their derivatives. These herbs have been proven to be safe and efficacious by long histories of practice, as well as by laboratory research done in China, Japan, Korea, and elsewhere. Now herbal tonics and preparations have been commonly accepted and widely used almost everywhere in the world. It is not difficult to find monographs describing Chinese herbal medicines in book stores, but in our opinion, this book may be the best one. Reading this book, you may become interested in the art of radiant health and begin to consume some Chinese tonic herbs or herbal preparations, which are of no harm to you and will soon benefit you if you select and use the herbs properly, as described in this book.

The art of radiant health was created and developed by the Chinese people. But it belongs to all human beings. We wish that these classical Chinese arts will be better recognized and used by all the people of the world, so as to improve both our health and our life.

—Xu Guo-Jun, Ph.D.
Wang Zheng-Tao, Ph.D.
and Zhou Zhen-He, Ph.D.

Xu Guo-Jun, Ph.D., professor emeritus at China Pharmaceutical University in Nanjing, China, is a member of the Advisory Panel on Medicine, Academic Degree Committee, China; member of the Consulting Specialist Committee (Pharmacy), Chinese Ministry of Health; director of the Chinese Pharmaceutical Association; and member of the Chinese Pharmacopeia Commission and the Chinese Academy of Sciences.

Wang Zheng-Tao, Ph.D., is a professor at China Pharmaceutical University, Department of Pharmacognosy; member of the Chinese Pharmacopoeia Commission; and director of the Chinese Academy of Medical Sciences' Commission to Standardize Chinese Herbs.

Zhou Zhen-He, Ph.D., is president of the College of Traditional Chinese Medicine at China Pharmaceutical University in Nanjing, China.

Introduction

We all want to live our lives fully, successfully, healthfully, and happily. In the Orient, these attainments are cumulatively called *radiant health*. Physical health by itself becomes irrelevant if it is accompanied by a troubled life, unhappiness, or failure. The loss of our physical health can become an all-consuming disaster. Sooner or later, most of us fall prey to various disharmonies in our lives and to small or serious ailments, which can accumulate and disrupt our lives and reduce our capacity to live fully or reach our potential.

Yet it *is* possible to build and protect our health so that we can live life optimally. Radiant health is attainable, and we can maintain it once we have it. This is possible when we learn the secrets of living in accord with nature's laws and take advantage of a few of nature's tools.

Among these great tools discovered by humankind to aid in the attainment of radiant health are the Chinese tonic herbs, also called the superior herbs. These tonic herbs are the elite members of the Chinese herbal system, the most fully developed herbal system in the world. The Chinese tonic herbs have always held a very special place in Asian culture. These very special natural substances have been associated with the highest qualities of living, and thus are associated with the ideals of long life, slow aging, glowing health, happiness, wisdom, physical vitality, adaptability, sexual vigor and response, mental acuity and clear intuition, love and compassion, and harmonious relations with nature and with one's fellow human beings. By achieving these goals, one can be said to have attained true radiant health.

The ultimate purpose of consuming Chinese tonic herbs and applying the principles of this way of radiant health is not so much to eradicate disease as to achieve these ideal goals of living. It has become clear over many centuries that the great Chinese tonic herbs can make a major contribution toward one's ultimate well-being by providing very special nutrients that help the body-mind become radiantly healthy.

What distinguishes Chinese herbalism from other systems has been the attitude the Chinese and other Asian societies have taken toward health. Putting the emphasis on *promoting* health, they have created a body of knowledge concerning the health-promoting tonic herbs matched by no other society or system, which have traditionally emphasized the remedial over the preventive.

The Chinese have chronicled their discoveries and passed the knowledge along from generation to generation for over three thousand years. Because of their respect for and continued utilization of these herbs, Asian societies have paid special attention to preserving these treasures of the earth. The vast traditional herbal knowledge has recently led to an intense search for scientific understanding and for new, improved methods of cultivation, production, distribution, and consumption.

As a result of three decades of research in thousands of institutions and laboratories throughout the world, Asian herbalism is now becoming well understood and is taking its rightful place as a major form of health care. Science and traditionalism have been well blended in Asia, where the traditional is respected but science is required to meet modern standards. Thousands of herbs have been thoroughly examined. Major research institutes throughout Asia have performed innumerable studies on the major tonic herbs, and thus these natural substances are now becoming quite well understood. There is a logic to the herbs based not only on age-old tradition but on good modern science.

THE EVOLUTION OF HEALTH CARE

Traditionally in the Orient, there were two main schools of thought concerning health care: the medical treatment (palliative) school and the health-promoting school, also known as the longevity school. The first emphasizes the use of various medical approaches to treat ailments after they have occurred, while the second stresses the benefits of developing superb health and promoting one's well-being, in order to prevent disease and increase the chances of a long and successful life.

In Asian societies, both approaches have always been blended, as they will undoubtedly be in Western society in the next century. But medical philosophy in the Orient is founded on the premise that the promotion of positive health is primary. Next in importance is prevention of specific disorders, followed by palliative medical care. An emphasis on the development of radiant health is the basis of tonic herbalism as well as other health-promoting systems in the Orient.

Modern, high-technology medicine has many wonderful benefits. It is truly extraordinary, and we can appreciate the level of knowledge and work that goes into developing new medical theories, techniques, and drugs. However, its emphasis on treating disease *after* an illness has occurred leaves a great void. It is becoming increasingly obvious that people cannot afford to rely on "medicine" to assure true health. We are deeply in need of a system of health care that encourages the *promotion* of health at all levels.

Most experts agree that in the next decade there will be a significant shift in the American medical system, which will now emphasize health-promotion techniques and preventive medicine. Individuals will be expected to take more responsibility for their own health and well-being, and the tools will become more available. Education concerning health matters will become more widespread, if not in schools, then by way of television, books, magazines, multimedia, and the Internet. This growing health awareness explains the huge growth in interest in physical fitness, nutrition, and dietary supplementation that has occurred in the past decade.

The shift has already begun to occur throughout our society. As they learn about the safety and benefits of most herbs, especially the Chinese tonic herbs, physicians are beginning to recommend them in situations that would have been unheard-of a decade ago. Tens of millions of people are now consuming the Chinese tonic herbs daily in America, Europe, Japan, and most other industrialized nations.

WHY I BECAME SO INTERESTED IN THE CHINESE TONIC HERBS

I believe that Chinese tonic herbs saved my life. They saved me where every other form of healing known to me at the time had failed. During my final year at the University of Michigan, I developed a severe case of chronic fatigue syndrome. Although I had been extremely athletic, my body broke down completely as a result of having burned the candle at both ends for too long. I had pushed my body's capacity to handle the stress of my lifestyle beyond the limit. I lost over fifty pounds and became so depressed that I contemplated suicide. I visited every doctor I could find but found no help. This went on for almost two years, and I grew increasingly despondent.

One day a friend gave me a bottle of a Chinese herbal tonic that he had recently purchased in Toronto's Chinatown called Shou Wu Chih. He didn't know what it was, but someone told him that it was a health tonic from mainland China that lots of students at the University of Toronto were taking because it gave them the energy to deal with the stress of school. That sounded pretty attractive to me, so I gladly accepted his gift.

The moment I drank it I felt that it was benefiting me. My instincts instantly told me it was good for me. I thought I could feel it in my cells (now I know that it was improving my circulation). About a week later I had in my possession a dozen bottles of this rich tonic elixir. In impressive style I started slugging it down—I didn't understand that you were supposed to dilute it. I finished off three bottles of Shou Wu Chih in a little over a week (that may not impress you now, but it will after you try it). It felt right—and it changed my life. I absorbed the tonics like a wilted plant fed a tonic solution of fish emulsion. By the end of that week, I was a new person. The veil was lifted, my energy came rushing back. The color returned to my skin and the dark rings under my eyes started to disappear. For the first time in nearly a year, I felt like running. I had found a miracle, and it formed the foundation of the rest of my life.

From that time forward, I dedicated my life to the exploration of the Eastern health care system and most particularly to Chinese tonic herbalism. A few years later I met my true teacher, Korean Daoist Master Sung Jin Park, who taught me the subtleties of the art of radiant health and of Asian tonic herbalism. From him I learned both the fundamental principles and many of the practical details of the ancient art that is as eminently applicable today as it has been for thousands of years. It is Master Park's teaching that forms the basis of mine.

THE TONIC HERBS
ARE TRANSFORMATIVE

Almost every person who uses the Chinese tonic herbs for any extended period of time will experience benefits. In some cases, as in mine, the benefits may be almost instantaneous and profound, while for others the influence may be subtle at first, with cumulative effects developing over time. My life had taken a very wrong turn, and by the law of vicious cycles my life was spinning out of control. One thing was leading to another, and eventually my health—and my life—would have become irretrievable. Instead, I was able to turn my life around, become healthy, and go on to enjoy a rich and fruitful life.

Indeed, one of the profound benefits of the Chinese tonic herbs resides in their ability to change "vicious cycles" to "benevolent cycles." The tonics help reverse the process of one problem leading to more problems. Something good happens when you start taking these herbs. You start to feel balanced and strong inside. You start having abundant energy when you need it and yet you feel relaxed and at peace. Incredibly, you become more and more adaptive so that you can do a lot of things that you couldn't do before. You find yourself taking on challenges you couldn't have handled before, doing things that you used to avoid or that you thought you were incapable of doing.

People start commenting on how bright your eyes are, how enthusiastic you are, how vibrant you are, how well you seem to handle problems, even how insightful you are. These are the *real* benefits of taking the Chinese tonic herbs. In many cases, the initial problems that led you to the herbs in the first place fade away and you forget about them as they become history, yet you continue using the herbs because they make you feel right, and your herbal knowledge becomes a major life asset.

Thus the vicious cycles we were experiencing are transformed into benevolent cycles. The Chinese tonic herbs are truly transformational. They are "growth herbs"—growth in terms of our character, our well-being, our evolution. They are transformative no matter what life path one is on. The changes may be subtle at first, but over time they become obvious. Success in whatever you do—that is the goal of taking the Chinese tonic herbs.

It is not necessary to become an herbal expert to take advantage of the tonic herbs. It is possible to achieve superb results by just knowing the basics and setting up a program that suits you. The more you know, of course, the more you can take advantage of the many extra benefits that the Chinese tonic herbs offer, but just gaining enough knowledge to develop and maintain your own program is sufficient. The system is so simple that even children understand it. All you need to do is learn the basic principles and study a few of the herbs and formulations and you're on your way. Then, if you are consistent, the benefits develop.

That is why I have written this book: to offer guidance in an art that will ultimately mean more to most of you than wealth—the art of radiant health. Of course, you must choose your herbs wisely and intelligently if you want to gain optimum benefit. Different tonics have different effects, and knowledge of these effects serves as a basis for selection. By familiarizing yourself with the Chinese tonic herbs, and the principles of Chinese tonic herbalism, you can make good choices and achieve maximum benefit from them. By the time you are done reading this book, you will be able to take full advantage of these great health products.

The potential for danger is minute. The tonic herbs are essentially foods. They are extremely safe and free of negative side effects. Side effects, if they do occur, are minor and generally self-limiting—they disappear as soon as you stop taking the herbs. If you take an herb that does not suit you, you might get gas or a stiff neck for a few hours. That's about it. However, it is always wise to be safe. Therefore, if you have any known medical problems, it is essential that you consult a qualified, knowledgeable health practitioner before trying the tonic herbs.

The world is at a crossroads. If the human race is to survive and the planet is to be brought back to health, we all need to cultivate our own personal health in conjunction with the health of human society and the health of the environment. As our collective awareness develops, it is becoming clear that our personal well-being is totally dependent upon the health, sanity, and well-being of human civilization and the health of the planet. Each of us, in our own way, can contribute to making this a better, healthier, more harmonious world—and live a better life as well. The Chinese tonic herbs can help sustain our physical, mental, emotional, and spiritual strength, necessary at this point in human evolution. But it all starts with you and me, and with our commitment to our own radiant health and that of our families and friends.

RADIANT HEALTH

CHAPTER 1

Attaining Radiant Health

THE ATTITUDE OF RADIANT HEALTH

One of the great secrets of a long, satisfying, and happy life, according to Eastern wisdom, is to focus on health instead of disease. This is the psychological basis of the art of radiant health. Develop the *attitude* of radiant health, and radiant health can be attained surprisingly easily. Once we have trained ourselves to focus on the attainment and maintenance of radiant health, and have acquired the tools for accomplishing our goal, the functions of the mind, body, and spirit can flourish. Once we have achieved a state of radiant health, the bodily functions cannot easily fall into disharmony, disease cannot readily arise, and, from the perspective of our physical, mental, emotional, and spiritual health, we are beyond most dangers.

Radiant health is attainable by most people who have not already severely damaged themselves through abuse and wrong living. It is also attainable by many who *have* severely damaged themselves but have the will to regain true health. In life, it is sometimes necessary to hit a low point before we discover the motivation to work at attaining radiant health. Complete success takes determination, knowledge, discipline, and skill.

But we cannot do it by ourselves. We need help. Nature can provide that help. One of the ultimate sources of help from nature lies in the nutritional resources. The tonic herbs, being one of the richest sources of bionutrients, are used to promote overall well-being, to enhance the body's energy, and to regulate bodily and psychic functioning, resulting in radiant health.

HEALTH BEYOND DANGER

Radiant health, the highest level of health a person can attain, is defined as "health beyond danger." In other words, the person is so internally strong and adaptive as to be able to adapt to virtually all normal stresses, as well as many extreme stresses, and is thus capable of overcoming most serious dangers. My teacher, Sung Jin Park, emphasized that *protection* is one of the primary characteristics of health, and the higher the level of protection the better. When one's protection has reached the stage of "health beyond danger," then one has achieved radiant health.

There are many Chinese tonic herbs that strengthen the body's resistance. Thousands of active components in the various herbs influence the human immune system. In particular, the tonics are rich in substances that "modulate," or regulate, the immune system. Regular consumption of a major immune-modulating herb, or a collection of herbs with modulating capacity, gradually builds up a person's resistance. I have seen hundreds of people who were immune deficient and thus prone to chronic colds and other infections. After taking the tonics for several months, their immune systems showed tremendous improvement. After taking the herbs for a year or so, they became highly resistant to common colds and flus. People find it amazing. It's this kind of response to the herbs that makes me think that the tonics are really foods that the body *requires*. It seems that without the herbs, the immune system is underfed. With the herbs in the diet, the immune system flourishes.

The combination of factors found in the tonic herbs makes them an indispensable nutritional requirement. They replenish Primal Essence, they provide the energy to adapt to the stresses in our environment, and they protect us. They can even strengthen our willpower. Radiant health is much more easily attainable if we are truly nourished, and these great tonic herbs provide a form of nourishment found only rarely in nature.

ATTAINING LONGEVITY

In Asia, longevity is universally regarded as one of life's primary goals. People do many things to assure their longevity. They work at an even pace, they eat three meals a day at very regular times, they exercise in a way that is believed to promote longevity, and so on. One of the measurements most often cited in determining the advanced state of a country is the average longevity of its citizens. The average life expectancy of a Japanese woman, for example, is eighty-six years. This is an astounding and wonderful achievement.

It would do all of us well to start thinking about longevity as a virtue rather than an inevitable catastrophe. It is possible to live long and to live well. If youthfulness is so important (which it is to me), then we should attempt to maintain our youthful condition into old age. By watching our health and promoting our well-being on a steady basis, we can reach old age without undue suffering. This does not in any way have to mitigate the excitement of life. On the contrary, with energy, protection, and intelligence, our lives will ultimately turn out to be richer and more exciting. And then the latter years of our lives can be truly great if we are not suffering from various ailments. While we are still young, it is wise to seek radiant health so that we can live a long, healthy, exciting, and happy life.

Wisdom is something that can grow as we grow older, so we should seek to learn the underlying truths of life as we proceed through life. We in the West would do well to respect the wisdom of older souls who have seen and done more than we have and who have the wisdom to understand what has happened.

My wife, who is Chinese, was very surprised when she first came to America to find out that there is not a single real, universally recognized symbol for longevity in our culture. Our Western culture seems to downplay the beauty of achieving great longevity. Youth seems to be king here. Yet we all eventually come to realize that life is finite and that growing old in a state of radiant health is far superior to living fast, hard, and foolishly while we are young and then suffering intolerable illnesses when we reach middle age and beyond.

In China and other Eastern societies, there are many symbols of longevity. You find them everywhere in China, Japan, Korea, and Southeast Asia, and they are used in a multitude of settings. Interestingly, an herb now commonly used in Chinese tonic herbalism is the most widely used symbol of longevity—the Reishi mushroom. This mushroom is used in all Asian societies as a symbol of health, happiness, wisdom, and long life. It is a common symbol in the art of China and Korea.

The Reishi is in fact a true longevity herb. Though historically it has been a rare herb, it has in recent years become much more commonly available, thanks to modern horticultural technology. Hundreds of scientific studies have confirmed that Reishi can be used to build physical resistance to disease and to treat a wide range of ailments. Reishi has many benefits, including protection of the cardiovascular system and prevention and treatment of liver diseases and even certain forms of cancer. No wonder it became a symbol of longevity.

We are fortunate today to have herbs like the Reishi mushroom accessible to us. There are many other similarly beneficial herbs that were once rare but are now easily obtainable. It is unfortunate that most people in the West do not even know that these herbs exist. When consumed over a period of time, these herbs can profoundly enhance the performance of our bodies and minds and can help us attain both radiant health and longevity. When used properly, they are completely safe and have no side effects at all. They are far less expensive than modern medical procedures used to cure illnesses and can be obtained at a local herb shop or health food store or by mail order.

HUMAN POTENTIAL POTENTIATORS

The Chinese call these tonic herbs "mild" because they are so safe and because they are not "druglike." They are not bolts of lightning, nor are they mind-altering in the same sense as we have come to think of drugs. But they are extremely powerful. When taken regularly for a period of time, we change. A whole host of functions tends to improve, we feel better and stronger, and we become more capable: more capable at work, more capable at home, more capable at play, more capable in bed, more capable in our art, more capable in every aspect of our lives. Our minds become clearer. We get more work done, and at a higher level. We look better and become more attractive.

The Chinese tonic herbs are so right for the age we live in. They are natural, they are effective, they are legal, and they are readily available. They can help us achieve what we want out of life. If we want energy, they can provide it. If we want willpower, they can help. If we need to relax, they can help us to calm down and loosen up. If we require endurance, they are truly effective. If we seek wisdom, they are a godsend. And if we want it all, why not? The Chinese tonic herbs are truly that good. Three thousand years of experience has proved that the Chinese tonic herbs are the virtual fountain of life.

The tonic herbs were considered by Daoist and Chan (Zen) Buddhist masters, who contributed heavily to the development of the art of tonic herbalism and to the art of radiant health, to be "spiritual growth herbs." The tonic herbs have been used for thousands of years by wise men and women and spiritual seekers to aid in their spiritual development. The herbs are not psychoactive substances like drugs. They are beyond that. Because they have profound regulatory functions that help the body-mind maintain its equilibrium even under extremely stressful circumstances, they are enormously useful in supporting our ability to overcome intense challenges and to learn from our experiences and thus to attain wisdom that might elude those less fortunate. The spiritual path is arduous and fraught with traps. And one of the biggest problems is that you may not even know when you are caught in a trap. The illusory nature of traps is legendary. Many spiritual seekers have used the superior herbs to clarify their awareness and put things in perspective. Ginseng, Reishi, and other similar herbs have played an enormous role in the spiritual world of Asia.

ADAPTABILITY:
THE MEASURE OF YOUR LIFE

The psychic power bestowed upon us by taking these herbs need not be the exclusive possession of the spiritually minded. The adaptive energy provided by the tonic herbs helps those who are not specifically on a "spiritual path" in a similar way. For one thing, the tonics help people handle stress much more easily. Success in the modern world can often be measured by how well we can handle stress. Those who handle stress well generally move up in the world much more quickly, taking on greater challenges, heavier workloads, and more confrontation, and in general getting more done. Successfully overcoming obstacles is the truest way to grow in experience, knowledge, and wisdom—all very good things. It could easily be said that the motto of our age is: "He or she who can handle more stress most successfully wins!"

Resilience is a significant aspect of radiant health. It results from adaptability, and thus the concept of adaptability is central to the concept of radiant health.

The ability to adapt to the stresses of life is fundamental to life itself. Adaptability is the root of evolution and the secret to biological success. The more adaptable one is, the more flexibility and resiliency one will be capable of showing in one's life. Adaptability is inherent in all living creatures, and human beings are inherently one of the most adaptable creatures on earth. They have been able to adapt to virtually every climate. There are humans living in the most inhospitable climates: the hottest, driest desert; the hottest, dampest jungle; the coldest, most barren tundra. But humans are now creating a new, often artificial world that is in many ways a new challenge to their adaptive nature. Not only is the well-being of every individual now at stake, but the very survival of *Homo sapiens* and the majority of other species is at risk because of extreme changes in the ecosystem resulting from aggressive technological "advancement."

It is not quite clear whether or not people are under more or less stress than they were in the past. Poverty, seasonal weather changes (without heating, insulation, or air conditioners), the hard work of acquiring food, war, pestilence, and so forth have always been stressful. Many of the stresses that our forefathers had to bear have been lessened by modern invention. What would we do without electricity, the modern toilet, the automobile, the telephone, the modern printing press, refrigeration, heating oil, grocery stores? On the other hand, life is so full of trivial pursuits and is so fast-paced that new stresses have arisen and we are being forced to adapt in new ways. Will we be able to adapt to the widening holes in the stratosphere? Will we be able to adapt to the carcinogens in our water, food, and air? Will we be able to adapt to artificial food? Will we be able to adapt to the constant bombardment of various forms of radiation?

A healthy person adapts easily to a wide range of "normal" stress factors, such as changes in the weather. But if for some reason we lose some of our ability to adapt, we can easily become imbalanced, and this often results in illness. And it is important to remember that an overreaction is just as dangerous as an underreaction. To be considered optimally adaptive, one must adapt precisely according to the degree of change.

If for some reason we lose the ability to adjust appropriately, sooner or later we fall prey to the forces of nature. In a desperate attempt to regain homeostasis, our bodies rely on backup methods of regaining balance. If these, too, are insufficient, severe symptoms arise, followed by death.

As the great endocrinologist Hans Selye has pointed out in his classic biomedical text, *Stress:* "Adaptability is probably the most distinctive characteristic of life. In maintaining the independence and individuality of natural units, none of the great forces on inanimate matter are as successful as that alertness and adaptability to change which we designate as life—and the loss of which is death. Indeed there is perhaps even a certain parallelism between the degree of aliveness and the extent of adaptability in every animal—and man."

Selye postulated that there is some sort of intrinsic energy with which a person is born. He presented compelling evidence that it can be used slowly or quickly, but when it is all gone, we die.

Adaptability is the very measure by which an Oriental master would judge the true health of an individual. The more adaptive an individual, and the more vigor with which one can meet the challenges of life, the greater that person's degree of health. The Daoist sages of China have taught that each of us is born with an intrinsic energy that determines our fundamental, constitutional strength. It is called Primal Essence, or *jing*. *Jing* is said to determine our potential life expectancy as well as the vitality of our life while we are living it.

Oriental sages say that it is easy to abuse and thus dissipate this *jing* with which we are born. As we lose this fundamental energy, we stiffen and lose our ability to change. We cannot adapt easily or appropriately, on either the microscopic or the macroscopic level. Therefore, we easily become imbalanced, toxic, and stagnant, dangerously susceptible to attack by microbial invaders. Selye has supported this principle of an original, apparently limited energy by demonstrating scientifically that stress of any sort can be adjusted to for a while, but that finally the stress-response mechanism exhausts itself and death ensues prematurely.

Long ago, Chinese sages knew this. They investigated the natural world, and over many centuries they discovered and developed means of enhancing this Primal Essence by working with the natural laws rather than against them. The oldest philosophical teaching of China, Daoism, is a philosophy of flowing with nature's changes, constantly harmonizing, always maintaining balance so as to avoid the stress of extremes. Nature itself presents enough difficulties. Why add more stress by bringing it upon ourselves? By knowing when you have gone far enough and by knowing when you have had enough, you will lead a less stressed, less draining life. Additionally, by living close to nature and by changing gracefully with the changes in the environment, you can avoid calamity and slow down aging.

Aside from simply avoiding stress, the ancient masters found it possible to *replenish* our reserves of *jing*. It is obviously impossible to avoid stress entirely. Anything that taxes our system drains us of some of our *jing*. Thus, to promote our health, we must nurture our *jing*—that is, our primal energy. Techniques were established to do exactly this, and have been passed along from one generation to the next for three millennia. These health arts for replacing spent *jing*—or beyond that, building reserves—are the greatest health secrets of the East.

Chinese tonic herbalism is a primary means in the Orient for replenishing and enhancing energy and for preserving harmonious balance in the human body. It is the primary tool for attaining radiant health.

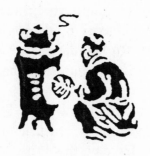

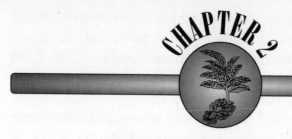

The Principles of the
Chinese Art of Radiant Health

ONENESS WITH NATURE

In the Orient, all philosophy, art, and science are traditionally based on the fundamental realization that there is an intrinsic unity to all things. All things and all processes are connected, and all things and processes influence everything else. The ancient Chinese thought of the world as a great mysterious ecosystem in which the health and vitality of one aspect of the system could be felt throughout the whole. They emphasized this unity and stressed that the glue that holds it together is the harmony of the system. Certainly, small disharmonies arise in nature, but they are immediately counterbalanced. If a change is radical enough, however, then the whole entity must change.

We can see this clearly today as modern man alters the face of the earth in amazingly broad strokes. Industrialization has so far resulted in ecological destruction. There are millions of examples, but one should suffice to provide illustration. We invent refrigeration, but the coolant is not fully understood in terms of its long-term effects on the environment. After just a few decades of use, it turns out that it is contributing to a depletion of the earth's ozone layer, which protects us from extraterrestrial radiation. As a result, animals and fauna are dying and humans are more prone to cancer and probably other disorders.

The human body, mind, and spirit form one complete whole within themselves and with the environment and the universe. Oriental philosophers and scholars long ago recognized the interconnectedness of the various parts of the body. Oriental knowledge of these connections is both extensive and enlightening. The organs have reflex actions on distant places in the body because of energetic, chemical, neurological, and psychic connections.

In the Oriental health arts, it is accepted as indisputable truth that the physical body and the psychic aspects of a human being are inseparable. Changes in one's physical being will result in changes in one's thinking and in one's intuitive and unconscious psychic processes. The state of one's mind likewise directly and indirectly influences the gross and subtle condition of one's physical nature. This notion of the interconnectedness of the body and the psyche is fundamental to the Oriental health arts.

Virtually all aspects of health and sickness are rooted in the union and disintegration of the body and the psyche. In the East, it is taught that by cultivating one's body, one can influence the quality of thought and intuitive experience, which can lead to a truly successful, happy, enlightened life. This is the basis of Superior Herbalism, the dietary and exercise arts, and acupuncture and acupressure. Conversely, cultivating the various aspects of one's psyche can and does have profound influence upon one's physical nature. This is the basis of meditation, guided imagery, and visualization techniques.

The Oriental health-maintenance and health-promotion arts, such as Superior Herbalism, take full advantage of this oneness of body and psyche to help each person grow to as full a state of health, well-being, and spiritual awareness as the person is ready to achieve. The tonic herbs are used to bring about changes in one's physical condition and are simultaneously used to influence the conscious and subconscious mind, the emotions, and the human spirit.

No form of health care is complete unless it recognizes and utilizes this principle of the unity of physical and psychic energy, because in fact there is no real distinction between them. Thus the goal of Chinese tonic herbalism is never to influence a singular change in just one aspect of a person's physical or psychic life. The real goal is to help the user of the tonic herbs to establish a harmony of body, mind, and spirit which can result in a new level of well-being, a new level of health and happiness that forms the foundation for true spiritual discovery, growth, and eventual enlightenment.

The principle goes beyond unity just within the isolated human being. A person is also always seen to be intimately interconnected with his or her environment in both the small and the large sense. Oriental philosophy is essentially naturalistic and recognizes that a human being is as much a part of nature as any other being of this planet. We have evolved over millions of years by the process of adaptation. A human life is complex beyond our imagination, but this complexity has evolved so that we can survive and flourish within the environment found on earth at this time.

Any change in the environment influences us both physically and psychically. How we handle such changes, how we adapt to the stresses of life, will be the determining factor in our health and well-being. Conversely, as we change, the environment around us will be influenced and will reflect our changes. Thus it is true that by harmonizing one's environment, one harmonizes one's own life. And in harmonizing one's own life, one's environment will be brought into order.

The greatness of Oriental natural philosophy lies to a great degree in the subtlety and breadth of vision with regard to the interconnectedness of a human being and his or her environment. The seeker of radiant health recognizes such influences as seasonal change, the wind, heat, cold, dryness, moisture, and so on as fundamental causative factors in one's health as well as one's dis-ease.

The greatness of Chinese tonic herbalism lies in its "adaptogenic" quality; that is, the ability to enhance the body-mind's capacity to adapt *optimally* and *accurately* to changes in the environment. This adaptability allows us to lead a much richer, broader, more adventurous life. Another aspect of the greatness of tonic herbalism lies in its ability to harmonize the physical energies within the body and to harmonize the physical and psychic energies of a human being so as to increase optimum functioning.

THE PRINCIPLE OF *YIN* AND *YANG*

The principle of *yin* and *yang* is the fundamental concept of the Chinese health care system. It is an all-embracing concept that can be used to describe virtually all natural phenomena. This principle has withstood the test of time and stands today as arguably our greatest model of the universe.

Yin and *yang* are opposing components of one integrated whole. They are totally interdependent, interacting constantly so as to maintain the normality and integrity of the whole. One tends to dominate the other, but no total dominance is permanent, and eventually the other takes its turn as the dominant force. This interplay of opposing forces establishes the basis of all existence and all change.

The Chinese call the principle of *yin* and *yang* the Great Principle. The Great Principle describes the innately dynamic, polar, cyclic nature of everything in the universe. Although many people find the principle of *yin* and *yang* foreign at first, it is in fact a very simple concept to grasp—and extremely reasonable. Every thing and every process in nature can be seen as having a cyclic nature and thus governed by the Great Principle. Light and sound move in waves that are cyclic. The earth turns on its axis, resulting in endless cyclic manifestations here on earth.

Human sleeping/waking cycles, seasonal changes, and the millions of microscopic cycles that support these daily and seasonal changes are the result of the larger cycles in our solar system, galaxy, and supergalactic systems. Within our bodies, our hearts beat, our lungs breathe, our glands secrete hormones, and our bowels and bladders excrete waste *rhythmically*. Each eye dominates for several minutes at a time, rhythmically. Indeed, virtually every human function follows rhythmic (cyclic) patterns.

Yin and Yang Defined

These rhythms are described and explained by the Great Principle, the principle of *yin* and *yang*. But what are *yin* and *yang*? *Yin* is defined as that part of a cycle in which energy is being accumulated, assimilated, and stored for later use. *Yang* is defined as that part of a cycle in which energy is being expended in order to create a manifest action. Thus *yin* is often associated with rest, receptivity, and quietude, while *yang* is associated with action, expansion, and movement. *Yin* should not be thought of as the absence of *yang*. Nor should it be automatically associated with weakness. *Yin* is at the very core of existence. *Yin* is in fact the very substance of life, and it is absolutely essential to all functioning. *Yang*, on the other hand, is the functional aspect of any process and is also essential to life. *Yang* sometimes seems more obvious than the inward-manifesting *yin*, but there is no *yang* without *yin*.

In Chinese tonic herbalism, we utilize the principle of *yin* and *yang* constantly. Some herbs are activating, drying, warm, or hot: these are *yang*. And some of these herbs affect the body profoundly and fundamentally to build up the *yang* power of the body, mind, and spirit: these are the *yang* tonic herbs. On the other hand, herbs that are nourishing, moistening, cooling, or anti-inflammatory are said to be *yin* in nature, and those substances that nurture the fundamental reserves of the body, mind, and spirit are called *yin* tonics.

In the Western world, *yin* and *yang* are often associated with the female and male forces. This association has its value, but in many ways serves to confuse students of Oriental philosophy until a deep understanding has been attained. Relative to one another, the female is often said to be more *yin* than the male, which is generally more outgoing and is therefore more *yang*. The female is said to be receptive and nourishing, while the male is said to be aggressive and protective. However, it is easy to see that many women are more aggressive than many men. These women would be considered more *yang*. And there are most certainly passive men who are relatively more *yin* than even the average woman. *Yin* and *yang* is a concept of relativity, and each person must be looked at relatively. An aggressive person with a hot temper would be considered to have a *yang* nature irrespective of gender; and a cold, passive person would be considered relatively *yin* irrespective of gender. In order to establish a healthy, balanced physiology, a person who is dry (*yang*) will need to increase his or her fluids and blood (*yin*), and a person who has cold extremities will need to invigorate blood circulation (*yang*).

The relationship of *yin* and *yang* is never static. The two forces are always vying with one another for dominance. First one dominates, then the other in its appropriate time. Under normal circumstances, the interaction of the two forces will remain within well-defined limits. *Yin* provides sustenance for the *yang*, and the *yang* protects the *yin* while carrying out the functions of the being. Neither *yin* nor *yang* will normally go to such an extreme that its opposing force cannot recover. However, if for some reason *yin* or *yang* exceeds the limits normally inherent in the system, the self-regulatory mechanism breaks down and crisis ensues. Health is dependent upon the maintenance of the correct balance of *yin* and *yang* forces in the body and psyche. Neither *yin* nor *yang* should increase or decrease beyond normal limits. It is possible through the application of Chinese tonic herbalism to help the body-mind maintain its self-regulatory capacity, assuring optimum functioning and radiant health.

One's basic physical constitution plays a very important role in one's long-term health pattern. A person born with a dominance of *yang* energy is said to have a *"yang* constitution." These fundamentally *yang* people often tend to suffer from *yang* symptoms throughout much of their lives. Conversely, a person born with a *yin* constitution generally suffers from *yin* symptoms. *Yang* symptoms tend to be more acute and more dramatic, but also tend to be overcome more quickly, whereas *yin* symptoms tend to be chronic, mysterious, and difficult to correct. It is important to take a frank look at one's constitution and to come to an understanding of how it affects one's life as a whole. It is possible to alter one's constitution to some small but significant degree by the use of Chinese tonic herbs, diet, and breathing and exercise techniques such as those taught by the Daoist masters, and by stimulating certain acupoints regularly for an extended period of time. Knowing yourself is a key factor in establishing radiant health.

Yin-Yang Self-Analysis

In order to best take advantage of the Chinese tonic herbs, it is wise to determine your *yin-yang* balance. The following table provides a few of the markers that can help you to understand whether you have a *yin* or a *yang* constitution.

YIN-YANG SELF-ANALYSIS

Yang Constitution	*Yin* Constitution
Large bones and sturdy frame	Thin bones and frail frame
Aggressive nature	Passive nature
Ruddy complexion	Pale complexion
Easily angered, a fiery disposition	Not easily angered, a tendency toward fear, anxiety, or melancholy
Testosterone dominant	Low testosterone or estrogen dominant
Sexually aggressive	Sexually passive
Illnesses tend to be acute	Illnesses tend to be chronic

If you have more of a *yang* constitution, you will tend to take more risks and be more aggressive in life than someone with less *yang*. *Yang* people generally live fast lives and burn the candle at both ends, thinking themselves invincible, especially when young. They often burn themselves out, however, and suffer from acute illnesses and radical breakdowns. If you have a *yang* constitution, you need to consume *yin* tonic herbs in all their various aspects. *Yang* herbs may be consumed as well to sustain your *yang* nature, but only in conjunction with *yin* herbs and usually in only moderate quantities. *Yang* people generally do better when they consume "cool" herbs.

If you have more of a *yin* constitution, you will tend to be more passive and cautious. You will be aware of your frailty and will naturally shy away from dangers that you instinctively know could harm you. *Yin* people tend to develop chronic, lingering ailments, which often appear not as serious as the acute illnesses that *yang* people contract, but over time they can be severely draining and debilitating. *Yin* people need to take plenty of both *yin* and *yang* herbs. The *yin* herbs replenish the lost *yin* energy. The *yang* herbs are necessary to replace, in a sense, the *yang* energy that is not theirs by constitution. *Yin* people tend to do better with "warm" herbs.

Most people do well with a balanced blend of *yin* and *yang* herbs, only slightly balanced in one direction or another, based on their original constitution. In fact, we all need to nourish both *yin* and *yang* throughout life if we hope to achieve radiant health.

BALANCE

Life and health are sustained by maintaining balance, even as the environment changes. Whenever there is imbalance, there will be discomfort. On the other hand, the state of being known as "well-being" is really a state in which everything is in balance—a state of harmony in all aspects of one's life. And it is a state that is genuinely attainable, though it may take much practice, depth of understanding, and wisdom to attain and maintain it.

There is no question that we have to work at being in balance when we live in a modern society. It is easier to fall out of balance than to remain in balance. There are many aspects of our lives that need to be watched and maintained in order to remain truly healthy: our diet, elimination, exercise, love life, work life, meditation, and so on. One must bring one's whole life into balance by bringing such details into balance. Doing anything to an extreme is contrary to this basic premise of maintaining balance. If we eat too much, we will pay for it sooner or later; if we eat too little, we will likewise suffer. If we exercise too much, we become sore or injured and could even shorten our lives; if we exercise too little, we will suffer disorders that will likewise shorten our lives.

Oriental sages have always taught that moderation is the key to health, happiness, and longevity—that is, radiant health.

One of the tricks to attaining a balanced life is to simply avoid extremes. An extreme high is always countered by an equally drastic low. By moderating one's highs, one can moderate one's lows. By moderating one's desires and by moderating one's habits, it is possible to attain a dynamic balance in all aspects of one's life that leads to the state of genuine well-being, which is a state of comfort and satisfaction.

Certainly, I am not advocating a boring, nonadventurous life. It is possible to do everything you want to do—just maintain your balance at all times. Actually, this is one of the areas where the tonic herbs are most useful. The greater vitality and adaptability and the deeper reserves provided by the tonic herbs allow a person to live a much more dynamic life than one would be able to experience if energy was in short supply.

Moderation and balance are different things to different people. What is extreme for one person may be moderate for another. The levels of available energy, adaptability, and energy reserves are the determining factors. I have seen many people completely change their lives by using tonic herbs. Their energy increases and their courage and self-confidence increase with it. As a result, these people seem to take much bigger chances than they did before they were using the tonic herbs, and they accomplish more. They are protected in their pursuits by an increase in adaptive energy and can therefore get away with a lot more stress before the body and mind pay a penalty.

Generally, it takes most people many years, if not an entire lifetime (if ever), to learn the lessons of moderation and the overall art of balancing one's life. An acute awareness of balance, and thus the principle of *yin* and *yang*, is the source of true wisdom. There are those who come to understand the principle of balance at a young age, and it is these who establish their health for a long lifetime. Those who wait to establish balance in their lives generally come to suffer serious ailments that lead them to seek a way to overcome their problems. By using the tonic herbs, one can help achieve balance in all aspects of life at virtually any age.

Chinese tonic herbalism is specifically and directly aimed at helping a person to become more balanced and to maintain balance by enhancing adaptability. This is accomplished in many ways. It is done by relaxing tense muscles that are contracted due to excessive energy supplies to that muscle or muscle group, and by stimulating and tonifying weak muscles. It is also accomplished by improving the ability of each of the organs to function optimally and harmoniously as a unified system. The tonic herbs strengthen the ability of the body to produce energy, to defend itself, to cleanse itself, and to rejuvenate itself.

In summary, it must always remain clear to the Chinese tonic herbal practitioner that balance is absolutely central to every action we ever take and to the results we hope to achieve. This balance is of a dynamic nature, governed by the principle of *yin* and *yang*. Practitioners of this great art must seek to establish and maintain a dynamic balance in their own lives so that they reflect the principles of balance at all times and under all circumstances. Those who endeavor to follow the way of *yin* and *yang* will develop a power and subtlety in their lives that will result in amazing achievements.

THE THREE TREASURES

Through the interaction of *yin* and *yang*, energy is created. From the densest object to the subtlest vibration, the entire universe is composed, at its fundamental level, of energy. Chinese philosophy is founded on the energetic nature of all things. Things are not seen materially, but as ever-changing states of energy. This is the same idea expressed by modern physics, which understands that mass and energy are one and the same. The Chinese word for energy is *qi* (pronounced *chee*). *Qi* permeates all things in the universe and is the motivating force of all activity. An ancient Chinese philosophical classic states: "There is nothing between Heaven and Earth but Qi [energy] and Dao [the laws of the universe]. Dao itself is based on Qi. Everything in the Universe relies upon it. When the Qi is outside Heaven and Earth, it embraces them. When Qi is inside Heaven and Earth, it circulates through and sustains them. Planets depend on Qi for their brightness; weather is formed by it, and the seasons are caused by it. Man cannot stand outside of Qi. It supports him and permeates him as water is contained within the ocean."

Qi exists everywhere, even in a lowly rock. The atmosphere is full of *qi*, and the air is a primary source of *qi* for human beings. The earth provides *qi* to us in the form of food and herbs.

The nature of life is to extract *qi* from its environment and to transform it so as to live, to adapt, and to create more life. The more energy, or *qi,* that a living system can accumulate and utilize, the more success it will have as a living being. A less-than-adequate ability to extract *qi* from one's environment and/or an inability to utilize it efficiently will result in failure of the organism and death, and possibly extinction of the species.

It is the purpose of Oriental tonic herbalism to improve the absorption and utilization of *qi*, according to the laws of nature. It is possible through the consumption of certain herbs, and through the development of one's breathing, to influence the various aspects of *qi* within our systems and to establish harmonious functioning as a result.

Qi, however, is not all the same. After observing both nature and the human body over many centuries, the Daoists defined several levels of *qi* in living beings. This knowledge led to the quintessential theory of Chinese life philosophy, that of the Three Treasures.

In the Daoist tradition, which forms the foundation of the traditional Oriental healing and health-promoting arts, there are said to be Three Treasures that in effect constitute one's life. These are known as *jing, qi,* and *shen.* There are no exact translations for these terms into English, but they are generally translated as Essence, Vitality, and Spirit.

The ultimate goal of all of the Oriental healing and health-promoting arts is to cultivate, balance, and expand the Three Treasures. At the highest level of the Oriental healing arts, the practitioner is attempting to harmonize all aspects of one's being. This is accomplished by focusing one's attention on the Three Treasures.

The author's great teacher, Daoist Master Sung Jin Park, described the Three Treasures by comparing them to a burning candle. *Jing* is like the wax and wick, which are the substantial parts of the candle. They are made of material, which is essentially condensed energy. The flame of the lit candle is likened to *qi,* for this is the energetic activity of the candle, which eventually results in the burning out of the candle. The radiance given off by the flaming candle is *shen.* The larger the candle and the better the quality of the wax and wick, the steadier will be its flame and the longer the candle will last. The greater and steadier the flame, the greater and steadier the light given off. Master Park described the Three Treasures in some detail:

There are Three Treasures in the human body. These are known as *jing, qi* and *shen.* Of these three, only *qi* has received some recognition in the West so far. *Qi* is but one of the Three Treasures—the other two are equally wondrous.

Jing has been called the "superior ultimate" Treasure, though even in a healthy, radiant body, the quantity is small. *Jing* existed before the body existed, and this *jing* enters the body tissues and becomes the root of our body. When we keep *jing* within our body, our body can be vigorous. If a person cares for the cavity of *jing* [a space within the lower abdomen], and does not hurt it recklessly, it is very easy to enjoy a life of great longevity. Without *jing* energy, we cannot live.

Qi is the invisible life force which enables the body to think and perform voluntary movement. The power of *qi* can be seen in the power that enables a person to move and live. It can be seen in the movement of energy in the cosmos and in all other movements and changes. *Qi* circulates through the twelve meridians [the energy circuitry of the body] to nourish and preserve the inner organs.

Shen energy is similar to the English meaning of the words "mind" and "spirit." It is developed by the combination of *jing* and *qi* energy. When these two Treasures are in balance, the mind is strong, the spirit is great, the emotions are under control, and the body is strong and healthy. But it is very difficult to expect a sound mind to be cultivated without sound *jing* and *qi*. An old proverb says that a sound mind lives in a sound body. When cultivated, *shen* will bring peace of mind.

When we develop *jing*, we get a large amount of *qi* automatically. When we have a large amount of *qi*, we will also have strong *shen*, and we will become bright and glowing as a holy man.

Jing (Essence)

Jing is the first Treasure and is translated as "Essence." *Jing* is the primal energy of life. It is closely associated with our genetic potential and thus is intimately associated with the aging process. The quantity of *jing* determines both one's life span and the ultimate vitality of one's life.

At conception, the refined Essence, *jing*, of the mother and father merges and becomes one within the new fetal cell, and this new life takes up residence in the womb. This united Essence creates an energy that forms the foundation of the new human being's life. It is called prenatal *jing* (or original *jing*). During pregnancy, the fetus relies upon the mother to nurture and protect the original *jing*. However, at birth, the infant becomes independent of the mother's direct umbilical nourishment and begins to breathe and eat by its own power. After birth, the original *jing* becomes active and aids in the transformation of foods and thus in the production of energy. Original *jing* acts as the primary catalyst for all energy transformation in the body throughout one's lifetime, and it provides the fundamental life force that determines the life span and the innate vitality of the individual. A small amount of original *jing* is released constantly, and this is used by the body to maintain all its functions. This active *jing* is called postnatal *jing* but is commonly referred to simply as *jing*. Original *jing* and postnatal *jing* have a major determining influence over both the length and the quality of one's life.

Jing is the refined energy of the body and is said to be the root of our vitality. It is very concentrated energy. *Jing* provides the foundation for all activity and the reserves required to adapt to all the stresses encountered in life. *Jing* is stored in each of the five primary organs. It is essential to life. When it runs low, we are forced to tap into our original *jing* reserves, and our life force is severely diminished, causing the loss of our power to adapt. When original *jing* is depleted below a level required to survive, we die. Eventually, everyone runs out of original *jing* and thus everyone dies (at least physically).

It is considered extremely difficult to enhance the original *jing* after conception, although it is not at all difficult to deplete and weaken it, and thus to weaken and shorten one's life. The only way to strengthen the original *jing* is through specific highly sophisticated yogic techniques such as those developed by the Daoists and by consuming certain potent tonic herbs known as *jing* tonics. The purpose of taking *jing* tonic herbs is to maintain healthy levels of postnatal *jing*. If postnatal *jing* is maintained at sufficient levels, prenatal *jing* is used much more slowly and the aging process is slowed down.

Jing is stored for the whole body in the "Kidneys," one of the five primary organ systems in Chinese health philosophy. The Kidneys, according to Chinese physiology, include the reproductive organs, the brain, the skeleton, and the adrenal cortex. *Jing* is concentrated in the sperm and ova. It specifically controls the functions of the reproductive organs and their various substances and functions; the power and clarity of the mind; and the integrity of one's physical structure. *Jing* is largely associated these days with the hormones of the reproductive and adrenal glands. Strong *jing* energy in the Kidneys, so the Chinese say, will lead to a long and vigorous life, while a loss of *jing* will result in physical and mental degeneration and a shortening of life.

Jing is burned up in the body by life itself, but most especially by chronic and acute stress and excessive behavior, including overwork, excessive emotionalism, substance abuse, chronic pain or illness, and sexual excess (especially in men). Excessive menstrual patterns, pregnancy, and childbirth can result in a dramatic drain on the *jing* of women, especially middle-aged women.

If one is under perpetual or acute stress and the reserves of *jing* in the Kidneys are used up, the only backup is the original *jing*. Further stress will result in a depletion of this original *jing*, which will in turn result in an overall weakening and breakdown of the body, mind, and spirit, causing a shorter life, even if the stress is overcome. There is a great Chinese maxim that should never be forgotten: "It is all right to become fatigued, but never to become exhausted."

There will be no severe permanent consequences if one experiences some stress that requires utilizing some of the *jing* reserves; but if one *exhausts* the available supply of *jing* and is forced to utilize original *jing*, one will pay dearly indeed. This idea of avoiding extreme stress and thus avoiding the depleting of one's original *jing* while cultivating strong reserves of *jing* lies at the heart of many of the standard health practices of the Oriental masters.

The use of the Chinese tonic herbs, as well as breathing exercises and diet therapy, profoundly influences the manufacture and transformation of the life energy. It is possible, by cultivating our own energy and protecting our original *jing*, to enhance the energy that we pass on to our children. *Jing* is refined to an absolutely pure state in the reproductive glands, and it is this refined *jing* that energizes sperm and ova and provides the genetic potential of our offspring.

The vitality, happiness, and longevity of our children, and theirs, will depend to a very large degree upon the quality and vitality of this *jing*. Enhancing this *jing*, this Primal Essence, is one of the ultimate goals of life, whether we recognize it or not, for this is the determining factor in the survival of the species. Modern Western man has apparently not yet grasped the long-range results of the way we treat our bodies. It is time to take the bigger view of life and remember that what we do at one moment will have consequences far into the future. We start by refining our character, practicing moderation in all things, accumulating *qi*, cultivating *jing*, and protecting ourselves against the unnecessary loss of our *jing*.

There are special tonics that fortify *jing*, and these are found among the *yin* and *yang* tonics. These *jing* tonics are used to replace the spent energy and to build up large reserves for future use.

Qi (Vitality)

Qi is the second Treasure, and in the Three Treasures system it includes both energy and blood. Although *qi* may be defined as all energy, in the Three Treasures system it represents human vitality on an immediate basis. This *qi* is the aspect of our life that involves action, function, and thought. *Qi* is the source of our vitality. It nourishes and protects us. The *qi* that nourishes us is known as nutritive *qi*, and the *qi* that protects us is known as protective *qi*. Both are produced from food and air on a daily basis.

In the system of the Three Treasures, blood is considered to be a part of the *qi* component of our being. Blood is said to be produced from the food ingested after the *qi* has been extracted through the action of the "Spleen," another of the five primary organ systems. The red blood cells are said to be nutritive and are *yin*, while the white blood cells are protective and aggressive and are therefore *yang*.

Qi tonic herbs, composed of energy and/or blood tonics, increase our ability to function fully and adaptively as human beings. *Qi* is said to be produced as a result of the functions of the Spleen and "Lungs," another primary organ system. Therefore, *qi* tonics strengthen the digestive, assimilative, and respiratory functions. In addition, they have potent immune-potentiating activity.

Qi tonics increase the amount and improve the quality of the energy and blood flowing through our system. This increase in energy and blood results in an overall increase in physical and mental vitality.

Shen (Spirit)

Shen is the third Treasure. *Shen* is our spirit. It may also be translated as our "higher consciousness." This is ultimately the most important of the Three Treasures because it reflects our higher nature as human beings. Chinese masters say that *shen* is the all-embracing love that resides in our "Heart," a primary organ system. *Shen* is expressed as love, compassion, kindness, generosity, acceptance, forgiveness, and tolerance. It manifests as our wisdom and our ability to see all sides of all issues, our ability to rise above the world of right and wrong, good and bad, yours and mine, high and low, and so on. *Shen* is our higher knowledge that everything is one, even though nature manifests dualistically and cyclically, often obscuring our vision and creating illusion.

Shen is the spark of divinity within each human being. It is the spiritual radiance of a human being and is the ultimate and most refined level of energetics in the universe. It is associated with our awareness of and oneness with the Universal Infinite Being and is manifested in our own godliness. *Shen* is not considered to be an emotion, or even a state of mind. It presides over the emotions and manifests as all-encompassing compassion and nondiscriminating, nonjudgmental awareness. *Shen* manifests not only as our love and compassion but also as our mental and intuitive energy.

Zhuang Zi, one of China's greatest Daoist sages, once wrote:

When the shoe fits, the foot is forgotten.
When the belt fits, the belly is forgotten.
And when the Heart [*shen*] is right,
"For" and "against" are forgotten.

This passage expresses quite exquisitely an aspect of Chinese Daoist philosophy that is absolutely central to the attainment of health. Very simply, Zhuang Zi is saying that one cannot attain high spiritual levels until one has learned the art of balance. Those who seek true happiness must achieve balance in their lives. Imbalance is the source of stress that distracts *shen*'s attention away from its higher path. But when there is balance and harmony in one's life, then the Heart, or *shen*, has an opportunity to develop and attain a state of enlightened, all-embracing acceptance of things *as they really are*, transcending the notions of good and bad, right and wrong, for and against.

It is taught in Chinese philosophy that *shen* naturally rules our lives, but if we lose our emotional balance (which we all do), then the ego and the various emotions compete for dominance and *shen* withdraws and becomes hidden. Immoderate behavior is brought about by a lack of understanding of the laws of nature, which promotes selfishness. We develop addictions to particular egoistic attitudes and to the emotions that help manifest our egoistic goals. Anger, greed, fear, worry, sorrow, frustration, uncontrolled and excessive worldly joy, the perpetual seeking of pleasure in the things of this world of relativity and illusion, are all examples of the types of mental states that force *shen* into hiding, often for the duration of one's life. If *shen* is weak, then the person becomes ruled by emotions and passions and the true desires of *shen* are covered by the demands of the body and of the lower self. The person constantly craves excitement and novelty, but these things do not satisfy the Heart, and the person is frustrated, lonely, and depressed.

The great spiritual paths of the world have all attempted to teach their followers that it is necessary to temper excessive desires and imbalanced emotions so that *shen* can naturally regain its position as the ruler of our lives. The Chinese Daoists have long practiced a spiritual path that emphasizes living in harmony with nature. They have stressed the idea of living a balanced life that flows with the seasons and various cycles of life, constantly adapting to each situation so as to minimize stress and allow *shen* to rule unhindered by excessive desire. Living so closely with nature, the Daoist masters realized that the body, mind, and environment were one and that these need to be cultivated in such a way as to allow the process of spiritual growth to proceed most fluidly.

In fact, all activities are directed by *shen:* thinking, seeing, speaking, hearing, exercising, working, and loving are all functions of *shen*. In health, these activities are performed pleasantly and rhythmically, but in sickness we see changes in all the human functions and activities, and there is a lack of mental clarity, and actions become disturbed. *Jing* and *qi* support *shen*, and if they are wasted (dissipated), *shen* will suffer. If *shen* suffers, it becomes shaken and withdraws. When the emotions are not subordinate to *shen*, they strive for dominance among themselves. This struggle eventually affects the organs, and disharmony and disease follow. This is why moderation is regarded in the Orient as the supreme way of health, happiness, and longevity.

Herbal remedies are capable of helping with many problems. But unless they help to raise the level of consciousness of those who use them, they are doing little. For this reason, the true tonic herbalist is always striving to open up *shen* and discover the nature of *shen*.

There is a great, age-old method of developing *shen*. The way to develop *shen* is to *give*. By seeing the divine beauty in all things and thus becoming a channel of divine love, we can rise above the small egoistical motives that drive most people's lives. The reward for true giving is *shen*. It does not matter whether or not you are paid for your service, because it is what is in your Heart and what flows from it that determines how your *shen* will unfold. If you give all of your caring, love, and wisdom, and truly try to help in whatever way you can, your reward will be far greater than the financial reward of the moment.

Certain true *shen* tonic herbs encourage the opening up of *shen*. There are also *shen* "stabilizers" which help stabilize our emotions so that *shen* reemerges and rules our lives. The emotions are allowed to play themselves out, but not to dominate our lives and become obsessions or even addictions. *Shen* tonics have been used by the great sages of the Orient to help in their quest for enlightenment and harmony with God, nature, and all of humankind.

It is also necessary to develop *jing* and *qi* so that *shen* has a body to survive in and through which it may radiate. The Three

Treasures form the very core of all traditional Oriental healing and health maintenance, but are often overlooked today. To forget them is to forget the very basis of the Oriental healing arts. It is possible to practice the Oriental healing arts at many different levels. But only by working at the level of the Three Treasures can one be said to be working at the level of the masters.

The Three Treasures and the Chinese Tonic Herbs

Tonic herbs are categorized as *jing* (*yin* and/or *yang*), *qi* (*qi* and/or blood), and *shen* (opening and/or stabilizing) by virtue of which Treasure(s) they nourish and develop. It is the fact that certain herbs are capable of providing these Treasures to those who consume them that separates Chinese *tonic* herbalism from other forms of herbalism. Though many herbs have medicinal qualities and some provide nutrition, only a select number are true "superior herbs."

Applying the principle of the Three Treasures is the highest form of herbalism. In the Orient it is called the Superior Herbalism.

THE FIVE ELEMENTAL ENERGIES

Yin and *yang* describe the primary polar aspects (or forces) of an entity or process. However, *yin* and *yang* can be defined even more subtly in order to understand the exact degree or stage of *yin* or *yang* in a cyclical process. The Chinese thus further defined *yin* and *yang* so as to refine the Great Principle. In so doing they developed the Principle of the Transformation of the Five Elemental Energies.

Again, *yin* and *yang* can be seen as the two poles of a cycle. The *yin* is the withdrawing, storing, nutritive stage, and the *yang* is the expanding, exuberant, active stage. The *yin* phase can be further described as consisting of two major segments: the early *yin* phase and the late (or full-blown) *yin* phase. *Yang* can likewise be divided into early and late phases.

The seasons provide an example of this. The year can be divided into two main phases: the months during which the days become longer, lighter, and warmer (*yang*) and the months during which the days become shorter, darker, and colder (*yin*). Thus the half of the year starting at the autumnal equinox and running through the winter is *yin*, and the six months from spring through summer are *yang*. Fall is the beginning of *yin*, and winter is full-blown *yin*. The *yang* phase is likewise clearly divisible into spring and summer, spring being the beginning of the *yang* phase and summer being full-blown *yang*. Thus there are four cardinal phases to the yearly cycle. The same four phases can be seen in *all* cycles.

The early Chinese masters gave each phase a name. The early *yin* phase was called *Metal*, the late *yin* phase *Water*, the early *yang* phase *Wood*, and the late *yang* phase *Fire*. In a *daily* cycle, the morning (early *yang*) would be the Wood phase, the afternoon (late *yang*) would be the Fire phase, evening (early *yin*) would be the Metal phase, and late night (late *yin*) would be the Water phase.

These four are the cardinal phases, but there is another aspect that in Eastern philosophy is absolutely essential to the understanding of the system, and that is balance. Without balance in a system, it would soon fall apart. Thus the great sages described a fifth element, balance, and called it *Earth*. The Earth element represents the balance and harmony within a system that is actually responsible for the integrity of the system as a whole. Earth is in the center, representing the pivotal, balancing, unifying factor of the whole system. Earth should thus be present at all times, because the system should always be balanced, albeit *dynamically*.

The five elemental energies are traditionally diagrammed like this:

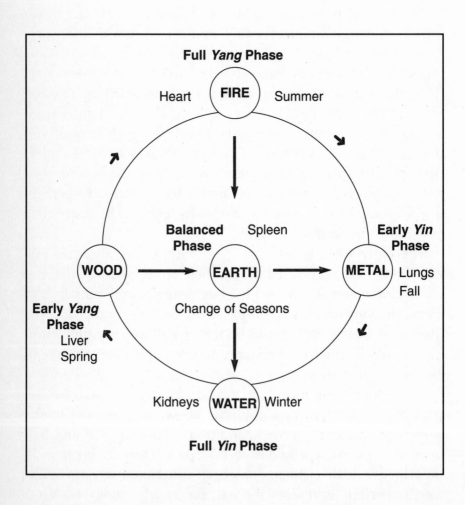

The Five Elemental Energies and Human Energetics

The five elemental energies also correspond to the various aspects of a human being, including specific organ systems, emotions, and sense organs. The following descriptions may provide some insight into the nature of each elemental energy as it influences the human condition.

WOOD

Wood is *new yang*—the first stage of a new cycle. It is an aggressive, vigorous energy that bursts forth from the depths of substance, expanding, invigorating all in its field of influence, bringing forth creation and life. Wood is the elemental energy of spring. It is associated with the "Liver," one of the primary organ systems.

The Wood element initiates activity. It is the creative urge and the procreative drive. It is the "will to become," the urge to grow and develop, to create our own existence. It is that which provokes and drives us. We experience it as the urge to express ourselves, to manifest, to break bonds, to metamorphose. We sense it as "spring fever." It is our will to open up, to expand. So when Wood is abundant, we develop, we create and procreate.

FIRE

Fire is the energy of growth to fullness, of full expansion, of warm, all-embracing love and compassion. Fire is the elemental energy of summer and is associated with the Heart. It is warm and full and has a fully developed *yang* nature.

When true Fire is unimpeded, life is joyous, exuberant, and loving, supported by courage, strength, and wisdom. Contentment, enduring vigor, a cooperative approach to life, clarity of understanding, and a free-giving spirit are signs of one whose Fire element is in proper harmony with the external being (the world and universe) and the internal being (the body-mind), which are in fact one. Feeling compassion, love, and joy without becoming overly excited, and giving of ourselves, are the natural ways to develop the Fire element.

EARTH

The Earth element is the energy of balance, of the center, and is thus always present. It is the pivot, or balancing point, of *yin* and *yang*. Earth is said to dominate at the change of seasons, during Indian summer, and during periods of atmospheric balance. It rules the Spleen energy system and directs the digestive system. It is experienced as a sensation of balance, centeredness, nonstriving, nonjudgmental contemplation, and sympathetic understanding. It is a mature energy, the energy of the ripening, well-adjusted soul.

Earth provides the energy of thought and reflection. It nourishes the flesh and builds strong muscles. Always seeing life from a broad perspective while remaining physically and emotionally centered will nurture the Earth element.

METAL

The Metal element is the energy of fall, and is thus the energy of retreat and withdrawal. It represents the transition of *yang* energy to *yin* energy. Metal controls the Lungs.

It manifests as an intuitive, contemplative sifting and letting go of that which is encumbering and useless to our inner life.

It manifests as the drawing within ourselves of that which is essential, that which is storable as concentrated energy, called Essence, and it is the active discarding of excess. It is thus analogous to harvesting, in which that which has grown in the previous *yang* season is collected, while the chaff, or useless by-product, is thrown away. It is the energy that draws life's forces toward us and deep into our body-mind for storage so as to ease the passage through the dark period soon to follow. It is the energy of release, freeing us of our old selves, outer attachments, and emotional entanglements.

WATER

The Water element is the energy of winter. Its power is very great, but highly concentrated. Water is associated with the Kidneys. It is the energy of the "seed," the fundamental energy of life which concentrates and matures deep within. It is indeed the very essence, the final distillation, of all accumulated energies and is thus very pure and of remarkable potential energy.

It is our "will to sustain ourselves," it is our courage. It is also our emergency reserve, the power of our mind, the root of our sexual vigor.

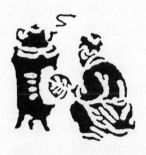

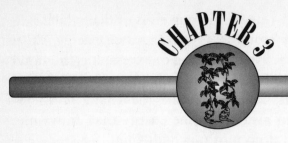

The Body–Mind from the Asian Perspective

THE CLASSICAL ASIAN VIEW OF THE HUMAN BODY-MIND

Chinese "organ theory" describes the body as an integrated, functional unit based on the production, circulation, and utilization of *qi*, in all its manifestations. According to the Chinese organ theory, there are five primary organs—Lungs, Kidneys, Liver, Heart, and Spleen—and each is related to one of the five elemental energies. These organs are really, by our modern standards, major functional systems. There is more emphasis in the traditional Chinese health system on the functional relationships of the organs than there is in Western medicine. The organs, as defined in the Chinese health care system, are not just the specific organs as we know them, but include whole systems of related functions, tissues, structures, emotions, and responses to the environment.

At first glance, an organ may not seem to be related to its

functions. For example, in Chinese health philosophy, the skin is considered to be a function of the Lung system. In the West, few people see the connection. Modern physiologists, however, recognize the close relationship between the lungs and the skin, both of which evolve from the same embryonic tissue and both of which have respiratory and eliminative functions. The Kidney system controls such functions as the reproductive system, mental clarity, hearing, hair, and the skeletal system. Again, modern physiologists can explain relationships between these functions based on neurological and hormonal interactions.

LEAKING *JING*

The five primary organs are all considered to be *yin* because they store *jing*. When functioning correctly, they do not "leak." All of the organs become more stable when they have an abundance of *yin jing* stored within their tissues.

However, these organs can "leak," and often do. "Leaking" in this case is defined as any loss of energy that should be stored. It is the job of the professional herbalist or practitioner to discover where energy is being leaked, determine why it is being leaked, to plug the leak, and to reestablish energy and functional balance in that organ. This is one of the primary secrets to becoming a master practitioner of the Chinese healing arts, and in particular to becoming a great herbalist.

There are many causes of leaks. An inflammation, for example, causes a serious leak of energy and resources from the body. It requires enormous energy on the part of the body to maintain an inflammatory response. Those with chronic inflammations die earlier than they would if they were inflammation-free. Recent studies, for example, have led scientists to conclude that as many as half of all heart attacks are the result of chronic inflammatory conditions in the major arteries near the heart. This is a new concept in the West, but one that makes perfect sense to all of us who have been involved in Chinese health care. Inflammation is called false fire in Chinese medicine. The Daoists have been teaching for over three thousand years that chronic false fire around the heart will ultimately result in heart failure, kidney failure, or both. Sung Jin Park, my teacher, explained that as we become older, the *yin jing* becomes weaker. This allows Heart *yang* to expand uncontrollably and attack the heart. This shortens life. To the Daoists, both Kidney *yin* (*yin jing*) and Heart *yin* must be maintained in order to control Heart *yang*. There are famous Heart tonic formulations that contain powerful yet safe anti-inflammatory herbs. These are among the most important longevity herbs of China.

THE ROOTS OF CHINESE PSYCHOLOGY

Perhaps the greatest distinction between Eastern and Western health philosophy is the way that the two systems handle psychology. Asian philosophy emphasizes the unity of body and mind, whereas Western philosophy has attempted to separate the body and mind to as great a degree as possible. The Chinese have always associated the emotions directly and intimately with the organs. They do not perceive the emotions as being stuck in the brain as we do in the West. Asian philosophers link the emotions to each organ and have developed incredibly deep theories of psychology based on these relationships. These theories are deeply engrained in Daoist and Buddhist philosophy.

In Chinese health philosophy, each organ system manifests a range of emotions. Thus the state of mind and the state of one's body are intimately connected. In the West, although it is understood that certain physiological conditions can influence the mind, mental and emotional disorders are generally not connected to specific organs or organic functions, but are believed to be wholly centered in the brain.

Fundamentally, the Chinese associated the emotions and related mental states to the five elements and to the organs associated with them. In general, the emotions are related to the organ associated with each element.

THE FIVE PRIMARY ORGAN SYSTEMS

It is critically important to free oneself of the *non*integrated way of perceiving the organs, as we normally view them in the Western world. When we speak of the Kidneys or of the Heart or the Lungs in the context of Oriental health philosophy, we are speaking of much more than the specific organs we know from Western physiology and anatomy. We are speaking of whole, highly integrated groups of functions and structures that form the very basis of our lives.

The following discussion of the five primary organs provides the basic functions normally associated with these organ systems in Asian health philosophy. By understanding these functions, it is possible to perceive the body, mind, and spirit as a whole and thus be able to penetrate the secrets of human health and disease. By making this knowledge part of life in a practical way, we can start on the road to radiant health.

THE LUNGS

The Lungs control physical energy

The Lungs control *qi*. By increasing and decreasing the rate and depth of respiration, one can control one's energy.

If the Lungs are weak, breathing is shallow, constricted, or otherwise weak and deficient. If the Lungs are strong and vital, the breathing is long, quiet, and deep, and the body fills with energy. The development of respiratory power and control is fundamental to radiant health. Regardless of the amount or quality of the food we consume, it will not energize the body if breathing is insufficient, just as a candle will not burn if there is no air available. Oriental masters insist that all sickness is connected in one way or another to insufficient breathing.

Through breathing we can master the emotions

There is a close connection between breathing and one's emotional state. The masters of every tradition in the Orient have always taught that through breath control we can master our emotions, an achievement that is basic to our health and happiness. However, if we have not developed the power to control our breathing, we will remain at the mercy of our lower selves.

When we are under stress or when problems arise, our emotions instantly influence how we breathe. For example,

- When we are angry, our breathing becomes rough.
- When we are worried or depressed, our breathing becomes shallow.

- When we are fearful, our breath becomes frozen.
- When we are in disagreement, we take short breaths.
- When we are frightened or surprised, the power of the breath goes into our inhalation.

Indeed, the emotions and breathing are one. The art of maintaining one's composure under stress, then, is accomplished through the practice of controlled deep breathing. Even when we become overwhelmed by anger or fear, or become depressed and sad, if the breathing is kept calm and long, then even the most powerful emotion will quickly subside.

The Lungs are the seat of wisdom

Wisdom is said to derive from the Lungs. Cosmologically, the Lungs are associated with the Metal element. The Metal element is associated with the ability to let go of the old while learning the lessons contained within experiences. Throughout life, we are required to face a never-ending set of circumstances from which we can learn the lessons of life. But many people become stuck in the emotion of the actual experience and instead of learning the lessons, become locked in the past. As emotions become habitual, they begin to rule our lives, and *shen* loses its power. In effect, we become addicted to certain emotional responses and respond throughout our lives like a broken record.

Deep breathing is the tool of the masters for letting go of old attachments and old emotions and for extracting the wisdom hidden within the experiences of life. In learning these lessons, we grow and evolve. Eventually, those who have learned the art of letting go and extracting the wisdom hidden within each experience will become profoundly wise. Thus the Lungs are said to be the seat of wisdom.

The Lungs control the skin

The skin has important respiratory functions in humans, just as it does in other animals. If there is an abundance of free-flowing *qi*, the skin opens and closes appropriately to adapt to changes in the weather.

Cosmetically, the Lungs have a profound influence over the skin. Any skin disorder, including blemishes and dry skin, is aided by balancing the Lung function and improving breathing. Lung tonic herbs are beneficial to the skin.

The Lungs produce the defensive energy, *wei qi*

The defensive energy, *wei qi*, produced by the Lungs is of critical importance to one's health. This energy is *yang* because it circulates at the surface of the body and supplies the skin with the energy to defend the body against climatic and pathogenic forces that could otherwise penetrate the body and cause damage to the internal organs. Thus the Lungs play a major role in the defense energy of the system. Lung tonic herbs play a major role in tonifying this defensive *qi*.

The Lungs affect the upper respiratory tract and voice

The functioning of the nose and sinuses is an important reflection of the health of the Lungs. If the Lung energy is flowing freely through the nose, the sinuses are clear, the nose is open, and the sense of smell is acute.

The voice reflects the state of the Lung energy. If the Lung energy is full and vital, the voice will be likewise strong, full, and clear. If the Lung energy is full, the speech will be easy and will not tire easily. If, on the other hand, the voice is weak and lacks any force, it is likely that the Lung energy is deficient.

THE KIDNEYS

The Kidneys, in Chinese health philosophy, constitute a complex organ system that includes much more than the renal function with which they are associated in the West. In the Oriental health philosophy, all disease can be traced to the Kidneys. It is always beneficial to regulate and strengthen the Kidneys, no matter what the disorder, and even when there is no disorder.

The Kidneys are the Root of Life

The Kidneys store and generate the fundamental life energy of the body and are considered to be the power source of our entire being. Like the root of a plant, the Kidneys are the deepest source of life energy to a human being, and our life depends upon the primal power contained in the Kidneys. Strong Kidneys will lead to a strong and long life.

There are *yin* and *yang* aspects to the Kidneys. The classics call the *yang* primal energy of the Kidneys *yang jing*. If this *yang* energy is weak, the body and the mind are depleted, weak, and dull. The *yin* primal energy is called *yin jing*. If the *yin jing* is depleted, the body degenerates and ages quickly. *Yang jing* is associated with the Fire element and *yin jing* with the Water element.

The *yang jing* is the primal energy source of the entire body throughout one's life. It generates all the *yang* energy of the body and motivates all the activities of the organs. Without it death would ensue. The *yang jing* keeps the body warm and generates, in particular, the activities of the mind, reproduction, and birth.

Because both *yang jing* and *yin jing* are located in the Kidneys, the Kidneys are said to be the root of *yin* and *yang* and of Water and Fire for the entire body. These two opposing primal forces constantly interact and together are called the Root of Life, which is the source of growth, transformation, regeneration, and reproduction. Neither one can exist without the other, and a deficiency of one or the other will lead to imbalances in other organ systems that will eventually cause disease and even death if the original imbalance in the Kidneys is not corrected.

The Kidneys store *jing*

The Kidneys are the great reservoir of energy for the entire body. This energy, *jing,* is stored in the Kidneys and can be released to any organ or to the whole system upon demand.

The Daoists have always taught (with great emphasis) that the secret to a long and healthy life is to accumulate an abundance of *jing* in the Kidneys and to avoid its reckless dissipation. This is accomplished by avoiding excessive and abusive activities in one's lifestyle, by avoiding stressful situations and emotional excess as much as possible, by breathing and exercising in such a manner as to accumulate energy and directing that energy to the Kidneys, and by eating foods and consuming tonic herbs that nourish the Kidneys and build *jing.*

Certain tonic herbs can actually provide *jing* directly to the Kidneys and their associated organs. That is why the Kidney tonic herbs are considered to be the primary antiaging and longevity herbs of Chinese herbalism.

The Kidneys control reproduction and fertility

When the *yang jing* rises, stimulating the Liver, sexual arousal occurs. If the *yang jing* is sufficiently strong, ejaculation of the seminal fluid will occur in the man, and the woman will excrete vaginal secretions and experience intense orgasm. This can result in impregnation if the woman is healthy and ovulating.

Fertility is generally associated with the *yin jing*, while potency is associated with *yang jing*. *Yin jing*, in this regard, represents the hormones and other substances and fluids related to reproductive functioning and fertility. The Kidneys control fertility.

The Kidneys control the skeleton

The skeleton and all tissues immediately related to it are controlled by the Kidneys. When the Kidney energy is strong, the bones will be strong. The bone tissue itself is considered to be *yang* and is therefore under the influence of *yang jing*. Anything that strengthens *yang jing* will strengthen the bones.

The ligaments, cartilage, and tendons are associated with *yang jing*, but also to some degree with *yin jing*. *Yang jing* adds strength to the joints, while *yin jing* adds flexibility and resilience. *Yang jing* promotes healing. *Yin jing* is anti-inflammatory. Excessive stress or other Kidney-depleting activities can weaken these connective and supportive tissues, resulting in joint disorders. Therefore, all the joints are directly under the influence of the Kidneys. When the Kidney energy is flourishing, the joints are supple and strong, free from pain, swelling, and inflammation.

In particular, the lumbar section of the spine and the knees are very closely associated with the Kidneys. When the Kidneys are full of energy, the back and knees are strong and flexible, but when the Kidneys are weak, these joints are very vulnerable.

The Kidneys support the marrow

The marrow, the material inside the bone, is responsible for the production of much of one's blood, including red blood cells and many white cells. The marrow tends to degenerate as we age, and by the time we reach middle age, most of our marrow has dried up. The Kidneys are responsible for marrow and for its functions. Nurturing the Kidney energy is believed to likewise nurture the marrow and thus increase one's energy and immune functions, and thus lead to a longer, healthier life.

The Kidneys nourish the teeth

The Kidneys are said to control our teeth. Strong Kidneys will generate strong teeth that are resistant to disease, decay, and breakage.

The Kidneys provide the vitality of the brain and mind

The brain is generally associated with the Kidneys. Kidney *qi* nourishes the brain tissue itself, and the mind is said to be energized by the Kidneys. Thus if one's Kidney energy is abundant, one's mind will be sharp and clear, memory will be powerful, and intuitive and cognitive powers will be great. On the other hand, if the Kidney *qi* is depleted, the mind will be cloudy and slow, memory will be weak, and intuition will be veiled. Forgetfulness and "spaciness" are usually treated by tonifying the Kidney *qi*.

Many yogic systems, including Daoist and Tantric Yoga, utilize special techniques for transforming Kidney (especially sexual) energy into psychic power. Tonifying the Kidneys will strengthen the mind. Overworking or otherwise exhausting the mind will deplete the Kidneys.

The Kidneys control hearing

The Kidneys control hearing, and thus acute hearing is a sign of strong Kidneys. Deafness, ringing in the ears, and other symptoms of impaired hearing are signs of weak Kidney energy.

The Kidneys control excretion and urination

Just as in Western physiology, the Kidney is said to control the excretion of urine. When the Kidneys are functioning properly, the body fluids are abundant and flow smoothly throughout the body. Constipation and difficult urination, however, may be signs of excessive Kidney fire or of water deficiency. If the Kidneys cannot transform water, urination is weak and the body swells, resulting in edema.

The Kidneys control the hair on the head

The hair on the head is controlled by the Kidneys. *Yin jing* deficiency and/or an excess of *yang jing* can result in excessive hair loss. Tonifying *yin jing* in particular can prevent or reverse hair loss. Premature graying of hair is also associated with stress-related depletion of the Kidney energy.

The Kidneys control our healing energy

The energy that we use up in the process of healing ourselves and others is the Kidney energy. As practitioners of the Oriental healing arts, it is absolutely essential to remember this, because if we give up too much of our own energy in the healing work we do, we are shortening our own lives. It is therefore necessary to constantly beware of the need to replenish our Kidney energy, particularly the *yin jing*, lest we become "burned-out," losing our power to help others and cutting into our own life span.

The Kidneys give us will and courage

When the Kidneys are full of *qi*, the body and mind naturally feel a sense of self-confidence and courage. Then the will to live is strong and the future seems bright. We automatically sense that we have abundant reserves of energy and know that to a large degree we are safe.

If the Kidneys are weakened and depleted by stress or other factors, the body-mind senses this as well and becomes fearful and paranoid. We know that the reserves are short and that another emergency or depleting situation might cause permanent damage or even death. And from the opposite perspective, chronic fear will deplete the Kidneys, resulting in other signs and symptoms of Kidney deficiency.

The Kidneys astringe *qi* and fluids

One of the responsibilities of the Kidneys is to consolidate the energy and fluids and prevent their leaking from the system. Master Sung Jin Park believes that one of the cardinal secrets of longevity is to prevent virtually all unnecessary leaking of the Essence. Leaking manifests as urinary and seminal incontinence, excessive perspiration, and diarrhea. Excessive emotions and incessant talking are also considered to be leaks that drain the Kidneys or result from weak Kidneys.

The Kidneys *store*. By tonifying the Kidneys, we increase their power to store.

The Kidneys control the power of digestion

Although the Kidneys do not directly digest food, the *yang jing* of the Kidneys influences our ability to do so. If the *yang jing* is strong, we can completely digest our food, and even a little bit of food can generate significant energy. If the fire of the Kidneys is weak, our digestive function is weak; food thus goes through undigested and we derive little energy and blood from it.

THE LIVER

The Liver, like the Kidneys, is a complex organ system. Its functions include not only those of the liver as we know it physiologically in the West but also a number of other organic structures and functions that might seem unrelated at first glance but are in fact closely related functionally.

The Liver stores and purifies blood

When we are active, our blood circulates freely throughout the body, but when we are at rest, much of our blood returns to the liver and is stored there. While the blood is in the liver, it is purified and changed. The liver plays the major role of detoxifying the blood. Chemical toxins and metabolic by-products are separated from the blood in the liver and are either discharged through the bowels or stored in the liver where they cannot harm other tissues in the body. Of course, chronic consumption of toxic substances will severely damage the liver over time. Therefore, a major part of strengthening the liver and making it healthy is detoxifying the liver itself.

The Liver smoothes and regulates the flow of *qi*

The Liver is responsible for the smooth flow of *qi* through the body. It prevents stagnation and accumulation of *qi* in the internal organs and meridians. If the Liver is not functioning well in this respect, there is a tendency to bloating and congestion in the digestive tract. Other conditions that can arise from the inability of the liver to spread *qi* are muscular tension, poor circulation, headaches, cold hands and feet, and menstrual problems.

The Liver manifests as creativity, ambition, motivation, and the "will to become"

When the Liver is balanced, *qi* flows smoothly, and a person will naturally be able to express ideas creatively. Creativity itself is a manifestation of the Liver energy. Liver is associated with the Wood element, which is associated with expansive energy. Ambition and drive are also manifestations of the Liver energy. A person with a healthy Liver will have a well-balanced urge to grow and develop and will feel happily and energetically motivated. This is known in the Chinese lexicon as the "will to become." The will to become is the will to live and to evolve. Without it, one will become depressed and lethargic. Depression and lethargy are clear signs that the Liver is not functioning properly.

The creative energy of the Liver manifests most fully at the early stage of new cycles, when a person's energy is fully charged and the future seems unlimited. The "honeymoon" of a relationship is just such a period that would be governed by the energies of the Liver.

Anger damages the Liver

Blockage of the Liver energy usually stunts one's creativity or the ability to express it, and inability to express creativity results in frustration. Since our society forces many people to suppress much of their natural creativity, many people build up Liver tension and frustration. If this frustration builds, the energy eventually turns to anger and rage. It is very difficult to suppress anger, which is an explosively powerful emotion, and eventually anger will manifest in one way or another. Anger is not always, or even usually, directed at the cause of the anger. People most often vent their anger in directions that will put up little resistance.

Anger should not be suppressed, but it should not be allowed to grow out of control either. Uncontrolled venting of one's anger will further damage the Liver. By regulating the Liver energy, it is actually possible to dissipate and dissolve old anger and to rise above the things that generate anger. It is very important to regulate the Liver energy and to dissolve old anger and resentment, because carrying this emotional energy around distorts one's entire life.

Anger often results in what is known as restrained Liver *qi*, which will manifest as tightness in the ribs and cold hands and feet. The Liver does not allow the *qi* to spread smoothly, and thus the circulation to the hands and feet is insufficient.

Excessive ambition can also result in frustration and anger, damaging the Liver. In fact, excessive desire of any sort will result in frustration because, by the very nature of this world, desires beyond attainability will result in frustration and depression. For this reason, all the great spiritual traditions caution their followers against harboring excessive desire and ambition.

The Oriental people also consider the Liver to play an important role in one's courage. Although the Kidneys influence courage by providing the raw hormonal power, the Liver influences courage by generating animal desire along with the human capacity for intelligent planning and decision making.

The Liver controls the peripheral nervous system and regulates the degree of muscular tension

One of the great tricks to understanding the nature of the Liver function, as described in the Chinese healing arts, is to realize that the Liver function includes all the functions of the peripheral nervous system of the body. The peripheral nervous system includes all the nerves that emanate from the central nervous system, including the nerves that innervate the organs and tissues of the body, the arms and legs, the face, and the genitalia.

When the Liver energy is functioning properly, the energy flowing through the nervous system will flow smoothly. Blockage of this function, known as *qi* stagnation, results in muscular tension. This is an extremely important syndrome. If the Liver malfunctions, as when we are chronically frustrated or angry, or when the Liver is toxic, muscular tension results. This tension will manifest wherever there is weakness. So, for example, if the Lungs are out of balance, the tension will manifest along the Lung meridian and around the areas directly related to the Lungs and their functional accessory tissues. The same would be true for any of the organs.

Muscular tension often occurs most severely in the regions specifically controlled by the Liver and the Liver meridian. For example, it is always said that the Liver controls the neck. The main meridian of the Liver itself does not actually flow through the neck, but the gallbladder meridian does. The gallbladder is the *yang* partner of the Liver. If the Liver is tense or "heated," the gallbladder will become more *yang*, resulting in neck tension. This in turn can cause chronic or acute neck problems, jaw problems, and headaches. (The great majority of headaches are so-called gallbladder headaches, which are caused by blockage or suppression of the Liver's ability to express itself freely and satisfactorily.)

When the Liver fails to regulate the nervous system properly, the peripheral nervous system will become unruly. Spasms, cramps, twitching, dizziness, vertigo, convulsions, paralysis, and hypertension will result. Headaches, for example, are generally caused by spasms of the blood vessels and muscles of the head, neck, face, and eyes. This is a typical Liver symptom caused by an imbalance in the peripheral nervous system. Leg cramps, menstrual tension and cramps, back spasms, chronic shoulder tension, twitching, jaw tension (temporomandibular joint syndrome), muscular dystrophy, spastic colon, and so on are all manifestations of Liver dysfunction.

Conditions caused by this lack of control of the peripheral nervous system are known as internal wind conditions. Like the wind blowing, the energy shoots through the system chaotically and in bolts and waves. Drunkenness is a windy condition, and so are seizures.

The Liver opens into the eye and controls vision

The eyes are a part of the peripheral nervous system and are therefore controlled by the Liver. Both visual acuity and the condition of the eyes are under the influence of the Liver. Acute inflammatory eye diseases are generally associated with excess of Liver fire. Chronic eye disorders such as blurred vision, dizziness, dry eyes, and glaucoma are caused by blood and *yin* deficiency of the Liver (often in conjunction with *yin jing* deficiency). Anger and toxic substances will cause the eyes to become red, as will a lack of sleep, which harms the blood and *yin* of the Liver.

The Liver nourishes the tendons and ligaments

The tendons and ligaments are governed by the Liver, so when the Liver energy decreases, the tendons contract and become stiff, and movement is impaired. Liver diseases, due to diminished Liver energy, are often indicated by contracture, tendon soreness, curled tongue, and contraction of the scrotum. Excessive anger or chronically repressed anger and frustration will damage the Liver and cause the tendons to contract. Degeneration or injury to the tendons and ligaments is often a direct result of a weakened or damaged Liver. In general, the Liver and Kidneys play a joint role in maintaining strong skeletal integrity.

The Liver feeds the nails

The finger- and toenails are nourished by the Liver and provide an excellent indication of the condition of the Liver. Someone who has a healthy Liver function will have beautiful nails that are smooth, strong, and naturally shiny. If the Liver energy is depressed, the nails will be soft, thin, brittle, pale, dull, and ridged. There will also be a tendency to develop inflammatory conditions around them or chronic fungal diseases.

The Liver energy concentrates in the genital organs

The Liver meridian runs through the genitalia of both men and women and is thus responsible for male erection and female arousal. Sexual drive is closely related to the Liver's primary drive to create (procreate) and to manifest the future. Poor erection in a man or the inability to achieve arousal in a woman is the result of deficient Liver and Kidney energy.

The Liver benefits from calmness and smooth transitions

The Liver flourishes when transitions are smooth and general calm is maintained. Rapid, harsh change will damage the Liver.

Change is a form of wind, and wind stimulates the Liver. If the wind is excessive—in other words, the change is drastic—the Liver will not be able to make plans and have them carried out. The ability to make plans is an important function of the Liver, and the inability to do so can cause frustration and anger.

The Liver prefers to remain cool

The Liver is damaged by excessive heat and therefore prefers to remain cool. Excessive heat conditions can cause general hypersensitivity, allergic reactions, and the full range of Liver symptoms. The natural tendency of the Liver is to overheat, in which case the heat rises, causing neck tension, hypertension, bloodshot or inflamed eyes, headaches, and so forth. This is called Liver fire rising. Or the heat can dry up the Liver *yin*, causing Liver *yin* deficiency, which manifests as dizziness, depression, headache, irritability, blurred vision, nervous disorders, chronic eye problems, and menstrual difficulties. Hypertension, which falls into the pattern of these two syndromes (often a combination of both), is a major killer because it predisposes a person to severe cardiovascular incidents. It is treated by nurturing the Liver *yin* and quelling excessive Liver fire.

If, however, the heat combines with moisture, it can descend, resulting in inflammatory conditions in the "lower burner" (the pelvic basin). Urinary tract infections, genital inflammation, vaginal discharge, and other such inflammatory conditions are known as Liver fire descending with dampness, or simply as damp heat of the lower burner, and are treated by drying up the moisture and cooling the fire while balancing the Liver energy.

The Liver is the seat of happiness

Happiness is said to reside in, and emanate from, the Liver. Happiness occurs when there is no frustration and anger, and in the Orient this is closely associated with the idea of modifying one's desires and ambition so that frustration and anger do not become hidden within the Liver and destroy our lives. A balanced attitude will result in a healthy Liver and a calm and happy life.

THE HEART

Shen, the guiding spirit, resides within the Heart

The classics say: "The Heart is the Supreme Master of the organs and is the home of *shen*, the Spirit. If the Master is brilliant, his subjects are peaceful. If the Master is disturbed, his twelve officials [the body's organ systems] are endangered."

Shen is the spiritual aspect of a human being. *Shen* presides over the emotions, allowing them to manifest appropriately but overriding them when they are not appropriate. When *shen* rules, the oneness of all things becomes sublimely clear, and duality becomes an obvious illusion. One can see the whole picture—both sides of every issue and of every story. *Yin* is seen in *yang*, and *yang* is seen in *yin*. Good is seen in bad, and bad is seen in good. No dualistic position is absolute, and therefore tolerance, compassion, and patience become the guiding spirits of one's life.

When *shen* is "shaky" or "disturbed," any emotion can become dominant. Frequently, a person whose *shen* is disturbed will experience agitation, nervousness, heart palpitations, insomnia, dizziness and fainting spells, uncontrolled laughter and grief (often occurring only moments apart), hysteria, deep sadness, fright, and mumbling to oneself.

The Heart controls the cerebral cortex, consciousness, and the mind

The Heart function encompasses the cerebral function associated with the mind. The Heart therefore controls the mind and is capable of being the master of the body. The Heart maintains consciousness. The Heart maintains control over perception and thinking. Normal functioning of the Heart, as it governs the brain and mind, produces a clear, quick mind and a vigorous spirit.

The Heart controls the entire cardiovascular system

The Heart is responsible for the proper functioning of the entire vascular system, including the Heart itself. Both large and small blood vessels throughout the body are under the control of the Heart. The heart muscle is maintained by the energy of the Heart meridian and is protected by the pericardium. Blood obstruction of the cardiac tissue will result in angina pectoris, purplish lips, purple spots on the tongue, and shortness of breath.

Blood circulation is controlled by the Heart as well. This includes the capillary circulation as well as blood circulation through the large vessels. The pulse, which reflects the condition of one's circulation, is thus controlled by the Heart function.

The color of the face reflects the condition of the Heart. A bright red face indicates an excessive condition of the Heart. A pale, lusterless complexion indicates a deficient condition, and if it continues, the skin will become not only lusterless but dark, because of blood stagnation.

The tongue is the orifice of the Heart

The tip of the tongue also shows the condition of the Heart. If the tip of the tongue is bright red, this indicates excessive Heart fire, while a pale tongue indicates a deficiency of blood and Heart *qi*.

The entire tongue is said to be the orifice of the Heart, and therefore when the *shen* is disturbed, one cannot speak (as when one is in shock).

The Heart helps regulate blood pressure

If Heart *qi* is sufficient, blood pressure will be maintained at a proper level. If Heart *qi* becomes deficient, blood pressure may be low, the limbs will be cold, the tongue will be pale, and the pulse will be weak and may skip beats.

THE SPLEEN

The Spleen controls gastrointestinal functions and generates *qi*, blood, and bodily fluids

The function of the Spleen in the Chinese healing arts is different from that associated with the spleen in Western physiology.

For one thing, the Spleen function encompasses the various digestive and assimilative actions of the pancreas, stomach, duodenum, and small intestine. Therefore, the Spleen is most accurately associated with the gastrointestinal functions that generate *qi*, blood, and body fluids.

The Spleen, which is sometimes translated as the "Spleen-Pancreas," is in charge of the transformation of energy. It is the responsibility of the Spleen to transform food both chemically and energetically so that it can be utilized by the body. It is thus responsible for the various stages of digestion and assimilation, and especially for the extraction of *qi* from the food in the stomach and its transmission to the Lungs, where it is blended with the *qi* extracted from the air inhaled, thus creating the essential *qi*. If the Spleen is strong, the body will be strong. But if the Spleen is weak, it will be unable to extract energy from the food one eats, the body will be weak and frail, and the following symptoms are likely: congestion in the stomach and small intestines, lack of appetite, bloating and gurgling, anemia due to poor blood production, and reduced immune function.

The Spleen is also responsible for the distribution of the chemical, fluid, and energetic constituents of food to all the appropriate parts of the body. Therefore, it can be said that the Spleen is like the earth, which nourishes everything. The Spleen is thus classified as being of the Earth element. It is called the center, and being at the center is said to have a balancing and harmonizing effect on the whole body.

The Spleen controls fluid metabolism

Fluid metabolism is one of the very important functions of the Spleen. The classics say that swelling from excessive water is due to the Spleen function's being depressed. This is known as Spleen *qi* deficiency.

The Spleen is responsible for removing water from the digestive tract and for distributing it to the various tissues of the body for their own needs. But if the water stays in the stomach and is not absorbed because the Spleen is weak, there will be a tendency to watery stools, difficulty in urinating, abdominal bloating, and phlegm congestion. Edema, where the water stays under the skin and does not circulate properly, is also due to Spleen *qi* deficiency and is a major cause of chronic fatigue.

The Spleen maintains the organs in their proper positions

Gravity has a natural tendency over the years to cause the organs to sink. It is the Spleen's responsibility to provide energy to the muscles that hold the organs in their proper positions so that the organs do not prolapse (drop). The stomach, intestines, rectum, and uterus are especially vulnerable to prolapse, not to mention the general sagging of all tissues as one ages. Strengthening the Spleen function helps maintain the general *qi* so that over the years the organs and tissues stay vital and do not drop.

If a person is experiencing a prolapsed condition, such as hemorrhoids, hernia, prolapsed uterus, or varicose veins, it is necessary to strongly tonify *qi* by strengthening the Spleen function along with treatment specific to the disorder. In the Chinese healing arts, it should always be remembered that the underlying cause of a disorder *must* be discovered and corrected. It is generally also necessary to work at the more superficial level to deal with the specific ailment. But the tendency of many less mature practitioners of these arts, be they acupressurists, acupuncturists, or herbalists, is to try to "heal" the patient or client by concentrating on and eradicating the symptoms, or conditions that just underlie the symptoms. This cannot be done even with the Chinese herbs, acupuncture, or whatever. Prolapsed organs are an example of this. They cannot be truly corrected unless the underlying cause of the disorder, which in this case is *qi* deficiency due to a weak Spleen, is successfully addressed. In fact, it is important to go even deeper and try to discover if other organs, such as the Kidneys or Heart, have caused the Spleen to malfunction, and to discover what emotions or habits may be at the root of the problem.

The Spleen keeps the blood in the vessels

When the Spleen *qi* is sufficient, the blood vessels properly regulate the distribution of blood to all tissues of the body. The Spleen is said to regulate the permeability of the blood vessels, especially at the capillary level. If there is a Spleen *qi* deficiency, the blood vessels may leak, causing bleeding syndromes. Excessive menstrual bleeding and/or continuous bleeding and spotting between periods is often due to a Spleen *qi* deficiency and is treated by toning up the Spleen function. Another very common symptom usually associated with this important Spleen function is chronic bruising, which is often virtually spontaneous. Both of these syndromes are caused by a weakness in the capillary function, which is controlled by the Spleen. Other common symptoms are gastric and duodenal ulcers, hemorrhoids, and bloody stool.

Thus another primary responsibility of the Spleen is to maintain the volume of blood in the body. It does this by providing *qi* to the blood vessels and protecting them from collapse and from leaking and by regulating the production of blood from the food we eat.

The Spleen supports the immune system

The Spleen plays a very important role in maintaining the defenses of the body. It does this primarily by regulating the various constituents of the blood, which include the immune cells that defend the body against invading microbes. A deficiency of Spleen *qi* will result in chronic low-grade infections such as urinary infections or chronic colds. The specific location of the infection will depend upon which other organ functions are weak and vulnerable.

There is a tendency among Oriental therapists to try to treat only the function or organ system that shows signs of infection or inflammation. This is an insufficient approach. The *qi* and blood must be supported and the immune system enhanced by tonifying the Spleen *qi* in any case of reduced immunity.

The Spleen governs the muscles and the flesh

The quality and quantity of muscle and flesh are governed by the Spleen. If the Spleen is functioning well, the muscle will be full, well toned, and strong. If the Spleen *qi* is deficient, as a result of the poor production of energy and blood by the Spleen, there will be a tendency to become physically (muscularly) weak and fatigued. And because muscle mass tends to diminish, people with severe Spleen *qi* deficiency tend to become very thin and emaciated. The Spleen must be strengthened in all wasting diseases. For this reason, people who develop conditions such as diarrhea and dysentery, which are symptoms of a very weak Spleen, become extremely fatigued within days and begin to lose weight if the condition is not remedied quickly. Chronic digestive weakness will likewise result in chronic fatigue.

In a more positive sense, people who wish to build muscle need strong Spleen *qi*. Spleen tonic herbs are famous for strengthening and building muscle.

The Spleen is connected to the mouth and lips

The condition of the Spleen can be seen in the mouth and lips. If the Spleen is healthy, the lips will be full and radiant and their color will be rich. But if the Spleen is depleted, the lips will be pale, emaciated, and lifeless.

Furthermore, the Spleen provides the moisture to the tongue and produces saliva, the "precious fluid." Saliva is necessary for proper digestion of food, especially carbohydrates, and also regulates and protects the condition of the mouth. A deficiency of saliva is generally considered to be a sign of stomach *yin* deficiency, but the root cause of the deficiency lies in the Spleen's inability to properly control the production and distribution of fluid to the mouth.

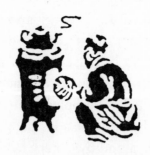

CHAPTER 4

The Superior Herbalism

THE THREE CLASSES OF HERBS

In the Orient, there are traditionally three categories of herbs—the superior, general, and inferior herbs. The superior herbs are health-promoting substances that have been found through centuries of use to improve overall health and resistance, increase energy, and lead to a long life. The general herbs are used to prevent specific diseases, or they can be used to provide the first course of action in case of an illness. The inferior herbs are specifically medicinal in nature and are used only in case of an illness.

These three levels were first described in the original classic of Chinese herbalism, attributed to the legendary emperor Shen Nong (the Divine Farmer) more than two thousand years ago. The following section from that classic explains the three levels of herbalism practiced in the Orient since that time.

> The INFERIOR CLASS of herbs are the assistants. They control the curing of illnesses and correspond to Earth. They possess a markedly medicinal effectiveness and must not be taken over a long period of time since side

effects will likely result. If you wish to remove cold, heat, and other evil influences from the body, to break up stagnation of any sort, and to cure illnesses, you should base your efforts on the herbs in the Inferior Class.

The GENERAL CLASS of herbs are the ministers. They control the preservation of the human nature and correspond to Man. One part of them possesses medicinal effectiveness, another part possesses preventive effectiveness. For every application, the choice of the suitable herbs should be considered carefully. If you wish to prevent illnesses and to balance depletions and consumption, you should base your efforts on herbs in the General Class.

The SUPERIOR CLASS of herbs are the rulers. They control the maintenance of life and correspond to Heaven. These herbs are not medicines, so the taking of these herbs in larger amounts or over a long period of time is not harmful. If you wish to take the material weight from the body, to supplement the energies and nutrients circulating in the body, and to prolong the years of life without aging, you should base your efforts on the herb foods of the Superior Class.

Of the several thousand herbs used in the Chinese herbal system, there is an elite group of fewer than a hundred known as the superior herbs, also called the tonics. The best-known and most important herbs associated with Asian herbalism fall into this category.

These superior herbs are not considered to be medicinal in the usual sense of the word. They are *not* used to treat specific disease or disorders. Herbs that are strictly medicinal fall into the inferior herb class because they often cause side effects and because they do not develop the Three Treasures. The tonics are used to promote overall well-being, to enhance the body's energy, and to regulate the bodily and psychic functioning so as to create what the Chinese call radiant health. The superior herbs provide this adaptive energy in abundance and are thus a primary source of true human empowerment.

Only herbs that meet specific qualifications are ranked as superior in the Chinese herbal system. For an herb to be recognized as a superior herb, it must have been found over many centuries to meet six specific qualifications:

1. A superior herb must contain at least one of the Three Treasures in such abundance that it can contribute to the building and maintenance of that Treasure in one who consumes it. Some of the tonic herbs contain just one of the Treasures, some contain two, and some contain all three. In other words, an herb must contain and be capable of providing *yin* (essential fluids), *yin jing, yang jing, qi,* blood, or *shen.*

2. A superior herb must aid in the attainment of a long life. By strengthening the life force, a tonic herb protects the body and provides it with a means of living out its genetic potential.

3. A superior herb must have broad and profound health-promoting actions that result in a radiantly healthy life. A tonic herb will in one way or another promote the functions of the body so that optimum health can be achieved.

4. A superior herb must have no negative side effects when used reasonably, and therefore may be taken continuously over a long period of time if desired, yielding cumulative, long-term benefits. This emphasis on safety is in accordance with the first law of Chinese herbalism—"Do no harm"—which is strictly adhered to by all practitioners of Chinese herbalism.

5. A superior herb must help balance one's emotional and psychic energy so as to help improve one's state of spiritual and emotional well-being and happiness.

6. A superior herb must taste good enough to be consumed fairly easily and must be easily digestible and assimilable when prepared correctly. Most of the herbs in the tonic category *do* taste good, and, in fact, most may be used in cooking. Many are used in a healthful Chinese diet and are considered by the Chinese to be a major food group. It is by virtue of the herbs' palatability that people have consumed them daily, generation after generation, for over three thousand years.

Of the thousands of herbs and foods tested by the people of Asia over many centuries, only a very small proportion have been determined to meet all these criteria. The superior herbs are the most prized of all herbs, for it has become clear that they can make a major contribution toward ultimate well-being. They can be consumed on a daily basis to fortify us for the adventure of life and to help us take full advantage of life's richness. Of course, in order to achieve radiant health, one must work on all aspects of one's life, but the tonics are considered to be an essential tool.

The superior herbs promote a long, healthy, vibrant, happy life, without any unwanted side effects even when taken over a long period of time. Essentially, these herbs are wonderful, healthful "superfoods" which benefit our well-being in ways that more common foods cannot. And they have a protective, balancing, vitalizing quality beyond that of any other herbs. They are generally consumed as a supplement to a well-balanced healthful diet for the purpose of completing our nutritional needs. However, these great tonic herbs have the capacity to promote health and well-being beyond that of other nutritional supplements. Regular consumption of the tonic herbs can and will provide a type of nutrition that is truly empowering.

The tonic approach emphasizes the use of the superior herbs and uses the general and inferior herbs only sparingly and only in a supportive manner, except when health irregularities or illnesses occur. By developing an understanding of the principles of natural health care, the way in which the body, mind, and spirit function, and the effects of the herbs, one can significantly improve one's health and promote a long, healthy, happy, satisfying, exuberant life.

These principles and the herbs that support the art of radiant health are easily learned, and herbal products are now available throughout the world in convenient forms that for the first time make it possible for anyone to take full advantage of them. Radiant health is in reach of most of those who seek it.

TONIC HERBS: THE FORGOTTEN NUTRITIONAL CATEGORY

Humankind evolved over millions of years by developing skills that allowed it to adapt appropriately and successfully to various and changing environments. Over those millions of years, humans relied on hunting and foraging, and much more recently on agriculture and horticulture. Early humans lived on a variety of foods that we would not recognize or understand today from a culinary perspective. A pot of stew ten thousand years ago most likely consisted of a rodent or other game cooked with a bunch of roots and barks collected within close range of the campsite.

Cooking played a critical role in our evolution. The discovery of cooking allowed primitive humans to significantly expand their diets. Soups and stews became possible, and a whole new world of edibles entered the human diet. In particular, many roots, barks, leaves, twigs, and other substances would simply have been impossible to consume without cooking. But once they could be made digestible, all of nature became primitive man's source of food and medicine. Undoubtedly, during this period, numerous herbs were discovered, and over centuries, and even millennia, knowledge expanded concerning the health benefits of various foods and herbs.

Thus in searching for food, primitive man discovered many medicinal substances. During the same period when agriculture was developing in China, herbal medicine was developing at a similar pace. In fact, the same legendary hero is considered to be the founder of both Chinese agriculture and Chinese medicine. Shen Nong, the Divine Farmer, was said to have discovered the techniques for farming and for healing with herbs. A book first published two thousand years ago, *The Divine Farmer's Classic of Herbalism*, is the oldest herbal text known in the world. Though it is attributed to Shen Nong, this classic was in fact the work of a large number of physicians and herbal masters compiled and written over many centuries. It is so remarkable because it presented an organized system of categorizing the herbs, a method that still makes sense and is still used today.

The Divine Farmer's Classic of Herbalism described 365 medicinal items, of which 252 were herbs, and the rest were of animal and mineral origin. The book divided these items into three classes. The first-grade substances, or superior herbs, were considered to be nourishing, strengthening, nontoxic, and suitable for long-term use—in other words, they were food-grade tonic herbs. The second- and third-grade herbs were clearly not food grade—they were distinctly medicinal. The second grade consisted of preventive, slightly harsh drugs. The third-grade items were very harsh drugs that the classic called the "poisons." It is clear that at that early time, human experience had already determined which plants, animals, and minerals were fundamentally safe to eat and which were not. The tonic herbs were considered absolutely safe. These first tonics would have been indistinguishable from food, since most food was still in a semi-wild state, even the cultivated variety. The Chinese have actually never lost that connection between food and medicine. There is an old Chinese saying that "medicine and food are of the same origin." And the connection between food and the tonic herbs has always remained so close that to this day in China you can order "tonic dishes" at most restaurants. These dishes consist of highly nutritious food with the addition of one or more major tonic herbs, such as Ginseng, Dang Gui, or Lycium.

To this very day, the Chinese believe that food is the best medicine and that the best medicine is herbal. Therefore, the Chinese consider herbs, and in particular the tonic herbs, to be an important food group used in healthy cooking. The tonic herbs have all of the same characteristics of excellent gourmet food, although not all of them are easily cultivated or easily consumed.

They should in fact be considered an essential component of our diet. They are highly nutritious, as safe as common foods, and in some cases are quite delicious. Unfortunately, many of them are not easily edible. Many are tough, fibrous, or woody. Siberian Ginseng, for example, is virtually a piece of wood. You would have to be a termite to eat it. But it extracts well in soup and tea. Another reason that herbs have been forgotten is their relative scarcity. Many of the tonic herbs only grew wild in mountains and they proved difficult or impossible to cultivate. Therefore, due to their rarity, they became very expensive and hard to obtain. Still, the Chinese obtain such tonics whenever they can and consume them as part of their diet.

In fact, only in the past century has our diet excluded wild vegetables and herbs. Until the modernization of our agriculture system, everybody consumed wild foods from time to time, if not daily. Just because foods of such high nutrition were rare or a bit difficult to prepare was no reason to cast them out of our diet and relegate them to the world of drugs.

Many of the foods we consider staples of our diet are important contributors of vitamins and other basic nutrients. However, due to the depletion of most of our soil and due to the industrialization of our farming, many of our vegetables have lost a great deal of their nutritional potency. That is why so many people are currently attracted to organically grown vegetables. And that is why so many people take vitamin supplements. But vitamin supplements alone are not even remotely capable of supplying all the nutrition that we require to attain and maintain radiant health.

It is time to realize that our society has forgotten an extremely valuable, if not invaluable, part of our diet. An herb like Astragalus Root, which builds the immune system and provides energy to our Lungs, is absolutely safe to consume daily. It should be as much a part of our diet as peas and carrots. When a person consumes it, his or her immune system says thank you. It seems to me that this is almost an essential food. It may not be essential in the sense that it is necessary to maintain life, but it is invaluable as a nutrient to support life at its fullest and most vibrant. There are a hundred other examples of herbs that should be considered food, members of the forgotten food group—the tonic herbs.

THE TONIC HERBS AS A PREMIUM SOURCE OF HEALTHFUL PHYTONUTRIENTS

For most of the past hundred years, nutritionists and other scientists have focused their attention on the vitamin, carbohydrate, amino acid, and mineral content of various foods. These fundamental nutritional substances have been thoroughly studied, though there is always room for improved understanding. More recently, the fiber, fat, and cholesterol contents of foods have attracted the attention of scientists because of discoveries concerning health benefits and risks associated with these substances.

However, only in the past few years has attention started to shift to a whole new range of nutritional components. A whole new category of substances called bionutrients has suddenly become the focus of much of the work and study being conducted by researchers around the world. The most common bionutrients are from the plant kingdom and are called phytonutrients.

Healthful, nutritious plants, so it seems, contain much more than vitamins and minerals, as important as these are. Tomatoes, broccoli, spinach, carrots, and most other vegetables contain hundreds of phytonutrients. Many of these phytonutrients have antiaging implications. Many build the immune system or improve circulatory functions. There are even quite a few that have been demonstrated to prevent cancer from developing.

As it turns out, Chinese tonic herbs, the herbs of Shen Nong's superior class, seem to be among the richest sources of phytonutrients in the world. They all contain dozens of phytonutrients that perform truly remarkable tasks in our bodies. We have just begun to explore the world of phytonutrients, but it is already clear that the tonic herbs are extraordinary sources of substances that can lead to radiant health.

ADAPTOGENIC ACTIVITIES OF THE CHINESE TONIC HERBS

The Chinese tonic herbs are broadly categorized as adaptogenic substances. An adaptogen is a substance that helps bring the body into a state of harmony with its environment by inducing chemical, cellular, and systemic balance. This harmonizing function reduces the effects of unfavorable conditions and stimulates the body's own immune and healing functions. These adaptogenic substances help the body to adapt to various stressful challenges presented by the environment and reduce the damage inflicted on the body. They tend to promote the body's own ability to cope successfully with stress, thus prolonging well-being.

Ginseng is considered to be the quintessential adaptogenic herb. Laboratory animals as well as humans that consume Ginseng have been found to adapt to dark and light more easily, handle high and low temperatures more easily, perform work more efficiently, and in general adapt to a wide range of stresses more effectively. Antifatigue activity has been demonstrated in both animals and humans. The mechanism by which Ginseng helps humans cope with stress is being intensively studied, but it is believed to be due to peripheral and neurogenic stimulation of the adrenal cortex, among other mechanisms. The adrenal cortex is part of the Kidney system described earlier. In other words, Ginseng helps tonify the Kidneys in such a way as to help protect the body during stress.

Numerous Chinese herbs are considered to be adaptogenic. Some of the better-known ones besides Ginseng are Siberian Ginseng (a distant relative of Ginseng), Gynostemma, Reishi mushroom (Ganoderma), and Schizandra. What is the basis for the adaptogenic activity found in the Chinese tonic herbs? Primarily, it is a characteristic called double-direction activity.

Double-Direction Activity of the Major Tonic Herbs

One of the qualities that distinguish the superior herbs from medicinal herbs and from drugs of all sorts is their remarkable ability to *regulate* body functions rather than force physiological activity in just one direction. Most of the great tonic herbs that have stood the test of time have this attribute. They help to establish and maintain homeostasis, which can be defined as normal, healthy body balance.

If a factor or set of factors causes certain functions to elevate, the healthy body normally possesses the ability to adapt in such a way that the function soon returns to a normal condition. For example, if someone is exposed to cold air, the body goes through a very complex process in order to maintain normal body temperature. If the body is exposed to hot air, the body goes through an equally complex process to keep the body temperature normal. If the body is deprived of oxygen, the body initiates a set of responses designed to increase oxygen consumption so that normal blood levels are maintained. If the body is exposed to excessive oxygen, mechanisms are invoked to slow down oxygen consumption. Certain factors that would cause our bodies to bloat are counteracted by physiological mechanisms that eliminate excess fluids. Similarly, factors that would cause us to become dehydrated stimulate us to consume and conserve fluids so as to maintain normal body conditions.

This type of regulatory activity takes place in thousands of ways every day, whether we notice it or not. The human body is a regulatory miracle.

Drugs and even medicinal herbs tend to stimulate a physiological activity in one direction only. For example, drugs designed to lower blood pressure must be monitored very carefully because they can drive blood pressure down too low. Diuretic herbs or drugs, if overused, can result in dehydration. This is the very nature of most drugs.

The Chinese tonic herbs work at a different level and in a different way. Remember that historically the superior herbs are not even considered medicinal, though when they are used, many conditions may be corrected. The superior herbs, the tonics, increase the vitality of the system as a whole. They strengthen the regulatory mechanisms of the body and mind in such a way that the body can maintain its balance even under severe duress. This is the secret of Chinese tonic herbalism. The tonics do not cure disease; they help the body to work the way that it was created to work—optimally, efficiently, accurately, and always with balance as the goal.

The Chinese were unique in developing a system based on herbs that tonify the deepest regulatory centers of the body. The Chinese herbs are loaded with antiaging, life-lengthening, pathogen- and cancer-fighting agents. But their most extraordinary ability is in helping to regulate the myriad of functions in the body so that the body and mind can remain youthful and radiantly healthy. Herbs like Ginseng, Siberian Ginseng, Reishi mushroom, Astragalus, and Schizandra, the stars of the Chinese tonic herbal system, have all been clearly demonstrated in laboratories and clinical tests around the world to have the ability to help the body regulate itself so that health is virtually locked in. That is where the Chinese got the idea of radiant health, "health beyond danger."

Siberian Ginseng, known as Acanthopanax in scientific circles, is a typical example of a superior herb with double-direction activity. For example, Acanthopanax prevents damage to various endocrine glands. In laboratory animals, it prevented adrenal hyperplasia due to ACTH, and reduced adrenal atrophy due to the administration of cortisone. In other words, it helps prevent both excess and deficiency conditions related to the all-important adrenal glands when forced out of balance by drugs. Similarly, it prevented thyroid enlargement due to the administration of thyroxin and prevented thyroid atrophy due to administration of methylthiouracil, a drug that normally causes atrophy of the thyroid. And again, it lowered blood glucose to normal in drug-induced hyperglycemic animals while increasing the blood glucose in insulin-induced hypoglycemic animals.

The Reishi mushroom, Ganoderma, an herb known in Asia as the Mushroom of Good Fortune is another of the premier superior herbs. It, too, has double-direction activity. It has been demonstrated to fortify the immune system when the immune system is weak or being attacked. It is used in Japan and China to treat many immune deficiency disorders including HIV infection and even some varieties of cancer. However, it is equally powerful at suppressing excessive immune response. Autoimmune diseases such as rheumatoid arthritis, many kinds of allergies, asthma, and lupus are routinely treated with Reishi in Japan and China.

If an herb does not have double-direction activity, it is a drug—an inferior herb. Herbs that have double-direction activity are extremely rare. Medicinals are much more abundant. No one will discount the greatness of drugs and medicinal herbs for emergencies and for acute conditions. But for chronic conditions and for establishing optimum health, it is essential that modern medicine come to recognize the profound beauty of the regulatory concept of double-direction activity.

THE IMMUNE SYSTEM AND THE CHINESE TONIC HERBS

Our immune system is a virtually miraculous network of activities designed over millions of years to protect us from viruses, bacteria, parasites, molds, dust, pollen, and malignant cells. It is the responsibility of the immune system to detect the intrusion, or invasion, of these entities and to mount a defense in order to eliminate them. A healthy immune system is capable of resisting most such intruders, and a very hardy system may be able to resist invasions that many other people's systems cannot.

If the immune system is weakened or malfunctioning, the invading microbes can easily establish a foothold in our body and disease sets in. Antibiotics can often be used to stop the invasion at this time, but chronic use of antibiotics further weakens the immune response. Furthermore, antibiotics are useless against viruses, pollens, and most parasites. They are certainly useless against malignant (cancerous) cells generated in our own bodies. It is much better to resist the invasion from within with a fully fortified immune system and not become ill in the first place. This is where herbs like Reishi are now attracting the attention of scientists and consumers alike.

Many chemical constituents play a role in Reishi's immune-modulating capacity. The polysaccharide components in particular seem to play an important role in attacking cancerous cells, but not healthy ones, while simultaneously strengthening the body's overall immune functions. The polysaccharides appear to help the body attack microbial invaders such as viruses, bacteria, and yeast. Scientific researchers have discovered numerous phytochemicals in Reishi that contribute to its immune-modulating capability.

Interestingly, many Chinese tonic herbs have been discovered to contain polysaccharides that boost the immune system—Astragalus, Codonopsis, and Ginseng, just to name a few. Research into the immune-boosting capacity of the Chinese tonic herbs is proceeding at a rapid pace around the world. Numerous phytochemicals are being discovered and are being patented by drug companies. Ultimately, however, the whole herb is what we want, and these are available to all of us.

ANTIOXIDANT ACTIVITIES OF THE CHINESE TONIC HERBS

The Chinese tonic herbs are among the richest sources of antioxidants. The vast majority of these herbs have now been shown to have significant antioxidant, free-radical scavenging activity. This antioxidant activity undoubtedly contributes to the overall action of these herbs as they promote health and well-being and prevent degenerative diseases. Many of the tonic herbs possess very potent antioxidant activity, far surpassing that of vitamins C or E.

Antioxidants are known to prevent and reduce inflammation, reduce the risk of cancer, prevent genetic mistakes, and slow down the aging process. A Chinese herbal formula containing many Chinese tonic herbs is likely to have dozens of antioxidants, all of which affect different tissues and functions in the body. Thus a Chinese tonic herbal formula is a broad-spectrum antioxidant.

The antioxidant activity in the body decreases with age, and it is no wonder that as we grow older the Chinese tonic herbs show more and more powerful rejuvenative benefits. In order to maintain our youthfulness and radiant health, it is essential that we consume a wide range of antioxidants virtually daily. The tonic herbs provide an incredibly wide range of these life-preserving phytonutrients.

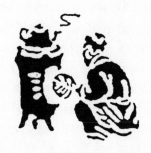

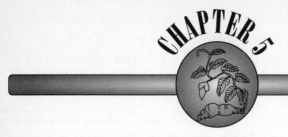

The Supertonic Herbs

The Chinese tonic herbs have been used through the centuries to promote radiant health. All of them are great herbs and all of them are commonly used today in China and elsewhere. But among the major tonics, there is an elite group of herbs that have been traditionally held in the most esteem for their capacity to promote radiant health. In order to put the tonic herbs in perspective, I have selected the herbs that belong in this elite group and have categorized them for our purposes as the "supertonics." I have selected twenty-two supertonic herbs based on their historical position in Chinese herbalism, because they have been shown by modern scientific research to be effective and safe, and because they are readily available in the American market.

It is important to know what the Chinese mean by the word "herb." Over the centuries, the people of Asia have tested virtually every conceivable substance for its nutritive, tonic, and medicinal qualities. The vast majority of foods and herbs are from wild vegetation, and most of the "herbs" used in Chinese tonic herbalism are in fact roots, leaves, flowers, and bark from plants. But Chinese herbalism has come to include more than just the plants of the earth. It contains sea plants, minerals, fish and other water-living creatures, special animal parts, animal by-products, insects, and all sorts of mushrooms. Chinese herbalism is not restricted to vegetarianism. This chapter and the one that follows, which describe the tonic herbs in detail, remain true to the reality of Chinese tonic herbalism as it is practiced around the world. A number of exotic substances will surely catch your attention. Deer Antler, Pearl, Gecko lizard tail, Royal Jelly (bee secretion—the food of the queen bee), Male Silk Moth, Placenta, Sea Horse, and other "strange" substances are described. Feel free not to use them if they do not appeal to you. They are included, however, because through the centuries these particular substances have proved to be profoundly beneficial to those who consume them. It is quite possible to eliminate all animal products from one's tonic herbal program, but I urge those of you who are not strict vegetarians to take advantage of some of the more exotic products.

THE FIVE CATEGORIES OF TONICS

There are five main categories within the superior class of Chinese herbs: energy tonics, blood tonics, *yin* tonics, *yang* tonics, and *shen* tonics.

Energy tonics, also known as *qi* tonics, increase physiological energy production. They are not necessarily stimulants, and in fact most are not. Instead, they help the body to function optimally, resulting in a natural increase in vitality. Energy tonics are generally believed to enhance the absorption of nutrients in the gastrointestinal system to yield energy and blood. Energy tonics that do this are said to influence the Spleen. Energy tonics also nurture the Lungs and enhance the extraction of energy from the air through the lungs into the body's energy system. *Qi* is then said to circulate throughout the body via the meridian system, providing the organs and tissues with the vitality required to live and function.

Blood tonics nourish the blood and help the body to utilize nutrients so as to function optimally. Blood tonics help build muscle and increase energy. Blood nourishes all the tissues of the body and provides the key means of distribution of nutrients, hormones, and immune cells throughout the body. Blood tonics are generally believed to benefit the quality and beauty of the skin. Women, who are often deficient in blood, often benefit greatly by regularly consuming blood tonics. In China it is said that "men are governed by *qi* and women are governed by blood." Men, of course, benefit from blood tonics as well. Some blood tonic herbs are also said to have "blood-vitalizing" activity. These blood vitalizers improve blood circulation.

Yin tonics nourish the fluids of the body and provide the "deep substance" of life. *Yin* and *yang* are the opposing forces within all systems. *Yin* is defined as the accumulation and storage of energy. *Yin* energy is generally condensed and stored in all of the tissues of the body, but most extensively in the major solid organs, and most particularly in the organs associated with the Kidneys. The stored energy, the energy considered to be the body's fundamental reserves, especially that stored in the Kidneys, is known as *yin jing*. The Kidneys, as described in Chinese herbalism, actually encompass the structures and functions of the reproductive system, the brain, the adrenal glands (especially the hormone-producing cortex), the ears, the hair on the head, the skeleton, the teeth, and the bone marrow. *Yin* tonics nurture these organs and functions. They also provide softness, coolness, and flexibility to the body and are necessary to healthy functioning. The *yin* tonics are usually associated with the preservation of life, and many of them are considered in the Orient to be the most important antiaging, longevity herbs.

Yang tonics are the power herbs of Chinese herbalism and, like the *yin* tonic herbs, are said to affect primarily the Kidney functions. *Yang* is the utilization of the *yin*, the stored energy. *Yang* tonics are generally said to have a "warm" or "hot" energy. *Yang* tonics are believed in China to build willpower and courage. *Yang* energy is also associated with mental creativity and the ability to manifest one's ideas. Certain *yang* tonic herbs are very famous as sexual tonics—some are even reputed in the Orient to be aphrodisiac, since *yang* energy is said to control sexual drive. *Yang* tonics build strength and are thus favorites of athletes. *Yang* herbs are used to stimulate metabolism, build muscle, and reduce the levels of fat in the system. They strengthen bone and are often used to strengthen the skeleton, in particular the back (especially the lower back), knees, and other joints.

Shen tonics allow for the development of *shen*, our Spirit. There are two categories of *shen* tonic herbs in the superior herb system: *shen* stabilizers and *shen*-developing herbs. *Shen* stabilizers calm and regulate the emotions so that *shen* can develop. *Shen*-developing herbs cause *shen* to rise up and to become prominent in our experience.

CATEGORIZATION AND RATING OF THE HERBS

When describing the tonic herbs, I will be using the following categories.

1. Pharmaceutical name: official scientific name used to describe the herb from a pharmaceutical perspective
2. Treasures: which of the Three Treasures are provided by this herb
3. Atmospheric energy: The herbs are said to have an energy that can be described in terms of temperature. Herbs are categorized as hot, warm, neutral, cool, and cold. Generally, hot and warm herbs are *yang*, while cool and cold herbs are *yin*. Neutral herbs are more balanced. This category is extremely important and is one of the key categories to remember when selecting herbs.

4. Taste: Each herb is said to have one of the five tastes, each taste associated with an elemental energy. The five tastes are: salty (Water element), sour (Wood), bitter (Fire), sweet (Earth), and pungent or spicy (Metal).
5. Organ associations: the organ(s) that the herb affects primarily
6. Qualities attributed to the herb
7. Varieties and grading: Herbs come in different varieties and grades. Slightly different varieties can have different chemistry and therefore different pharmacological effects. Better-quality herbs have been graded into different groups for the consumer. Most tonic herbs are graded according to the tradition of that herb. Higher-grade herbs are generally much more beneficial to the health and well-being of the consumer.
8. Preparation and utilization
9. Contraindications, if any

To put the value of these supertonic herbs in perspective, I have rated each of them, using a five-star rating system.

Treasure Rating	What It Indicates
None	The herb does not possess any of the Three Treasures, though it may have healing (medicinal) qualities.
★	The herb possesses a little tonic energy and thus tonifies at least one of the Three Treasures.
★★	The herb possesses enough of one of the Three Treasures to be considered a tonic herb.
★★★	The herb has real tonic power and should be considered for use in a tonic program.
★★★★	The herb is a powerhouse. It may contain a very large amount of one Treasure or large amounts of several Treasures. This herb is a supertonic.
★★★★★	This is the ultimate rating, reserved for the elite of the elite. An herb in this category is among the ultimate life-promoting substances ever discovered by mankind and should be considered by everyone interested in achieving longevity and radiant health.

It must be noted that the tonic herbs come in many grades. The ratings I have assigned are for the premium-quality specimens. Lower-grade specimens will have much less of the Three Treasures; in other words, they will have less *jing-, qi-,* and *shen*-developing capacity and will thus have proportionately lower Treasure ratings. For example, premium Ginseng, Reishi, or Astragalus may have a five-star rating, but lower-grade commercial varieties may have a rating of only one or two stars. That is why it is so important to understand *quality* and why it is so important to use only high-grade herbs from reliable sources.

THE TWENTY-TWO SUPERTONIC HERBS

There are dozens of tonic herbs that are tremendous life-supporting supplements. However, twenty-two of these stand out as the supertonics of Chinese herbalism. All of these are among the greatest herbs known to mankind. In this section, I will cover these supertonics in some detail.

Though it is difficult to say that one herb among this group is greater or more important than another, through the centuries a few of these herbs have acquired such reputations that they have become known to everyone who knows herbs. I have therefore chosen to present the herbs in roughly the order that I feel represents their importance in the Chinese tonic herbal system. All of these herbs, however, are true superstars and are incredible health agents.

GANODERMA

Pharmaceutical Name: Ganoderma

Treasures: *Jing, qi,* and *shen*

Atmospheric Energy: Neutral or slightly warm

Taste: Bitter

Organ Associations: Heart, Liver, Lungs, and Kidneys

Treasure Rating ★★★★★

Qualities Attributed to the Mushroom: Ganoderma, often called Reishi, has traditionally been used as an antiaging herb and has been used for many diseases and disorders as well. The health benefits of Reishi are extremely broad.

Ganoderma has double-direction activity. It significantly improves the functioning of the immune system whether the immune system is deficient or excessive. It is thus called an immune modulator. Reishi does not just "stimulate" the immune system. It *regulates* it. And that is what makes it so precious. If the immune system is excessive, as is the case with autoimmune diseases and allergies, Reishi can reduce the excess. A group of chemicals known as the ganoderic acids helps fight autoimmune diseases such as allergies. Ganoderic acids inhibit histamine release and improve oxygen utilization and liver functions. Ganoderic acids are also potent antioxidant free-radical scavengers.

Reishi is widely used in Asia to improve the cardiovascular system. It helps lower LDL (the "bad" cholesterol) and reduce excess fatty acids. It has been found to prevent and treat hardening of the arteries, angina, and shortness of breath associated with coronary heart disease.

It is an approved drug for some kinds of cancer in Japan and has been used safely and effectively, often in conjunction with other drugs or radiation. It has been demonstrated that Reishi can help reduce the side effects of many kinds of chemotherapy and radiation treatment and simultaneously contribute to the rebuilding of the immune system—an essential part of the recovery from cancer. Ganoderma stimulates the production of interferon and interleukin-1 and -2, which are potent natural anticancer substances produced in our own bodies. Reishi may well prove to be the greatest prevention against cancer because it helps us to protect ourselves by our own power.

It has also been approved in Japan and China for the treatment of myasthenia gravis, a serious autoimmune disease. Besides that, it is commonly prescribed in Japan for chronic bronchitis, memory loss, insomnia, hyperlipemia, and a whole range of degenerative diseases of the elderly, including disorders associated with senility.

Reishi is a superb antistress herb. It has routinely been used by mountain hermits, monks, Daoist adepts, and spiritual seekers throughout Asia because it was believed to help calm the mind, ease tension, strengthen the nerves, improve memory, sharpen concentration and focus, build willpower, and, as a result, help build wisdom. That is why it was called the Mushroom of Spiritual Potency by these seekers. Today, the people of Asia believe more than ever in Reishi's power to improve the quality of life by improving the inner life of a human being. All the scientific validation only explains the physical nature of Reishi, but it is the profound ability of Reishi to improve one's life on every plane that makes it such an incredibly beneficial tonic.

Everyone who takes Reishi notices the peacefulness that seems to accompany its use. Many people are able to stop using chemical drugs. And Reishi's effects seem to be cumulative, gradually strengthening the nerves and actually changing how we perceive life. Traditionally, Reishi has been considered to be the premier *shen* tonic of Chinese herbalism.

Reishi is indeed the "supreme protector," protecting us on every level—physically, immunologically, mentally, spiritually. It helps us adapt to the world and provides additional power for us to achieve a superior level of life. When we are so protected and so provided for, we can achieve things that would otherwise be impossible. That is why Reishi has been called the Herb of Good Fortune.

The primary constituents responsible for Ganoderma's medicinal actions are polysaccharides and triterpenes. More than a hundred different triterpene molecules have been identified in Ganoderma. Many other phytochemicals in Ganoderma may play a role in its health benefits. Constituent content varies among different strains of Ganoderma. Several triterpenes, not present in the mycelium, increase in concentration as the cap of the fruiting body develops. Quantitatively, the caps provide the richest source of triterpene acids, followed by the stem and then the spores.

Comparative constituent analysis was conducted on three strains of Reishi: red, purple, and black. The red and purple strains had similar triterpenoid patterns. The black contained little triterpenoid material.

Wild Ganoderma contains organic germanium, a substance widely believed, particularly in Japan, to have potent immune-strengthening and anticancer activity.

A derivative of Ganoderma strongly inhibited cholesterol synthesis. One mechanism of action is due to the ability of Ganoderma triterpenes to effectively inhibit the cholesterol biosynthesis pathway. Ninety-two patients with myocardial infarction and chest pain were treated with Ganoderma extract, and 72 percent of these patients felt the symptoms were relieved. Fourteen out of fifteen hyperlipemia patients treated with Ganoderma extract also showed decreased blood cholesterol levels. Numerous other studies have supported these findings.

Ganoderma has been found in numerous studies in Japan and China to reverse leukopenia, white blood cell death. It is widely used clinically in conjunction with chemotherapy to protect the white cells. The hot-water extract of Ganoderma showed the ability to activate natural killer-cell activity. The natural killer-cell activating factor is distributed in the fruit body of Ganoderma. Radiation protection can be obtained with administration of Reishi prior to irradiation.

The immunostimulant polysaccharides isolated from Ganoderma activate macrophages (a type of white blood cell), intensify phagocytosis, activate T lymphocytes (another type of white blood cell), and enhance cell-mediated immune response. The most immunologically active polysaccharides have an anticancer activity.

Japanese research has demonstrated that the extract of Ganoderma has an inhibitory action on histamine release from most cells. Therefore, it is potentially useful for Type I allergies, including anaphylactic shock, atopic dermatitis, hay fever, hives, drug allergies, and bronchial asthma. Ganoderma extract has also been shown to do well against such cell-mediated allergies as contact dermatitis and autoimmune disorders. The extract showed great enhancement of steroid-drug effect in the treatment of dermatitis. Due to steroid drugs' considerable side effects, any herb that can bring about a decrease in steroid dosage is beneficial to patients. The antiallergic activity of Ganoderma extract has been identified to be four triterpene ganoderic acids.

Ganoderma has been shown to have antihepatotoxic activity, to promote liver cell recovery after injury or surgery, and to be highly effective as a treatment for hepatitis.

Varieties and Grading: Shen Nong, the Divine Farmer, said that there are at least six varieties of Ganoderma. He noted red, purple, black, white, green, and yellow. Currently, one mainly finds Red and Black Reishi in herb shops. Occasionally, a Purple Reishi can be obtained, but usually not through normal channels. It is extremely rare.

Black Reishi, *Ganoderma sinensis,* is commonly available and can be found in most Chinese herb shops that carry bulk herbs. This variety is considered inferior, though it is certainly still a fine herbal tonic.

Wild Red Reishi is rare. This Reishi, which is the Reishi that Shen Nong was talking about, is much more potent and effective than the black variety. Red Reishi is *G. lucidum*, the primary Reishi. It is unlikely that you will find wild Red Reishi for sale in many herb shops in America, but there are a few superior products available that incorporate these mountain-collected mushrooms. The extraction yield from wild Red Reishi tends to be very low, so the extracted products tend to be more expensive. This is a sublime product.

Hothouse Reishi can be of good quality or poor quality, but most of it is poor. Reishi can now be grown in hothouses in a medium of sawdust and a nutrient such as rice. Most Reishi products sold in America are of the hothouse variety. They are inexpensive but not of high quality. The few superior sources of Hothouse Reishi available in America are from folks that have obtained special strains of Reishi from the Japanese scientists who first developed the modern strains of Red Reishi. Then they are grown in superior media. These mushrooms can even be obtained in their mycelial state from some mushroom mail-order houses, in which case you can grow your own fresh Reishi mushrooms. This is a real treat that I recommend very highly.

Reishi Mycelium: The mycelium is a whitish fungal blob that grows within a piece of wood or consumes some sort of nutrient until the nutrient is gone. At a certain time of year, the mycelium puts out its sexual apparatus, which is the mushroom that we see projecting out of the ground. Reishi mycelium was not traditionally used as a tonic herb by the Chinese or Japanese. However, it has recently been discovered that the mycelium is rich in the same polysaccharides that make the mushroom an effective health product, particularly as an immunostimulant. In fact, the mycelium has been found to contain much more polysaccharide than the mushroom, since the mycelium is much larger than the mushroom. This has led to many people using ground raw mycelium in products. These products usually do not include the mushroom. This has been widely accepted in America but not in China and Japan, where specialists argue that most research has been done on the mushroom, not the mycelium, and that the virtually miraculous health benefits of Reishi are found primarily in the mushroom. Though the mycelium may be useful, it does not match the efficacy and balance of the mushroom. Reishi mycelium is not a *shen* tonic, whereas the mushroom is the supreme *shen* tonic of Chinese herbalism.

Duanwood Reishi: The real deal, when it comes to Reishi mushrooms, lies in the domain of what is known as Duanwood Reishi, which is grown on certain specific varieties of wooden logs, without any chemicals, in a pristine mountain environment. In nature, Reishi grows on a large variety of trees in mountain forests throughout Asia. Just as "we are what we eat," a Reishi mushroom, too, is what it eats. Depending upon the kind of wood a Reishi grows upon, the Reishi may be powerful and medicinally marvelous, or it may be weak or even useless. The best Reishi grows on certain kinds of old hardwood trees that are indigenous to certain regions of China. The Chinese have made a thorough study of this, including years of pharmacological studies to determine which Reishi is the most potent, based on what kind of wood it is grown on.

The appropriate Duanwood trees are cut into short logs, usually about ten inches long. They are inoculated with Reishi spores and then planted in soil in mountainous regions of China. Growing Duanwood Reishi requires no pesticides or chemicals of any sort. In fact, chemicals ruin Reishi, so the government forbids it.

Duanwood Reishi is more than twice as potent as any other variety of Reishi mushroom available anywhere, with the possible exception of some wild Red Reishi. The Chinese and Japanese make extracts of it for injection and use it as a treatment for various forms of cancer. They also use it to treat hepatitis, arthritis, and other immunological dysfunctions. It is also sold as a premium, and rather expensive, tonic for domestic use in China and Japan, and more recently in America. Research has revealed the exact moment to harvest the Reishi to maximize the quantity and potency of the active constituents. These Reishi, however, should be used within one year of harvest or they lose much of their potency.

Reishi Spores have recently become a major source of interest in China and Japan. Reishi Spores contain huge quantities of polysaccharides and other ingredients that strengthen the immune system. The spores are now being used to treat liver and stomach cancer in China. As a health tonic, it is believed that the spores are even more potent than the mushroom cap itself. The spores, being seed, are believed to contain an abundance of *jing* and are therefore considered to be an antiaging substance. They are considered to be the virtual "elixir of life" to Asian herbalists. Spores are just now becoming commercially available in the West, albeit in small quantities and only through special sources. The spores must be purified, which is a difficult task because of their fineness. Traditionally, spores were believed not only to provide *jing* but to be the most subtle aspect of the Reishi, having a profound Shen-developing capability.

Preparation and Utilization: If you obtain a Reishi mushroom, boil it with other herbs for one to three hours. Slice it before you cook it. Never consume raw Reishi—it is useless, since it is very woody and not digestible. Most of you will consume commercially prepared Reishi. Find extracted brands made from high-quality Reishi. Consume it according to the instructions provided.

Contraindications: None. Although some people are allergic to mushrooms and other forms of fungi, the reported incidence of allergic responses to Reishi is virtually nil. Some people experience sleepiness when first taking large doses.

GINSENG

Pharmaceutical Name: Radix Panax Ginseng
Treasures: *Qi, shen,* and *jing*
Atmospheric Energy: Warm
Taste: Sweet and bitter
Organ Associations: Spleen and Lungs
Treasure Rating: ★★★★★

Qualities Attributed to Ginseng: On the basis of its pharmacological properties, Ginseng has been classified as an adaptogen. It is a powerful antistress agent. In Chinese health practice, there is a theory of *li qi*, which literally means "balance of energy." It is a term often used to describe the ability of Ginseng to balance the system at a fundamental level. In modern terms, this concept refers to the ability of Ginseng to help regulate body functions or to strengthen the functions that regulate other body functions.

Panax Ginseng is used by Chinese traditional doctors as a tonic for general weakness, poor appetite, low sex drive, shortness of breath, cold limbs, spontaneous sweating, and premature aging. Generally, Ginseng is used with other herbs. However, it is often used by itself.

Ginseng increases physical and mental efficiency and has been shown to improve the accuracy of work by promoting concentration. Ginseng prevents overfatigue. It is not a stimulant like amphetamines or caffeine, yet it increases alertness. However, it does not provoke subjective excitation (nervousness), nor does it disturb sleep. It is, in fact, used in a great many sleep-aid formulations. In China, there is an almost universal practice by high school and college students to chew several pieces a day while preparing for examinations and to chew it constantly during the examination period. Students claim that it makes them more alert, helps them stay awake for days on end with little sleep, and improves memory and reasoning ability.

Ginseng is a superb herb for aged people. It has a mental stimulant effect in elderly persons, improves memory and cognitive power, and can often reverse intellectual and mental deterioration. It quickens thinking and improves physical energy, often to a startling degree. Ginseng is very effective in hastening the recovery from illness and surgery.

The tonic benefits of Panax Ginseng are long-lasting. When Ginseng is taken for an extended period of time, the physiological changes that take place last for a long time after the Ginseng is discontinued (if it is discontinued). Studies indicate, for example, that increased work efficiency is retained from one to two months after a one-month course of Ginseng administration. People who take Ginseng to help regulate their blood sugar level will maintain normal blood sugar for several weeks after they discontinue Ginseng.

The main active constituents of Ginseng are its saponins, known as ginsenosides. Thirty-six ginsenosides have been isolated and identified from Panax Ginseng cultivated in the northeast of China. Panax Ginseng contains the following phytochemical constituents:

1. Panaxin and several related compounds, which act generally as stimulants to the midbrain, the heart, and the blood vessels
2. Panax acid, which is a stimulant for the heart and general metabolism
3. Panaquilin, which acts as a stimulant for internal secretions
4. Panacen and other volatile oils, which stimulate the central nervous system
5. Ginsenin, which lowers blood sugar
6. Vitamins A, B_1, B_2, and C

7. Bio-organic germanium (Ge), which is a powerful immunostimulant
8. A glycoside fraction that has been demonstrated to possess significant antioxidant activity

In general, the pharmacological action of Ginseng is dependent not only on its own constituents but on the condition of the organism consuming it. Ginseng shows double-direction activity at virtually every level of its action. This is undoubtedly why it has become so highly revered as a tonic and medicinal herb. It is also the basis of its classification as an adaptogenic substance. There are hundreds of examples of Ginseng's double-direction, adaptogenic action. Numerous studies have shown, for example, that it elevates blood pressure in cases of hypotension or shock, but restores blood pressure to a normal level in cases of hypertension. It normalizes white blood cell counts in cases of either excess or deficient white cell counts.

Even short-term administration of Panax Ginseng increases the adaptability of the organism consuming it. Numerous studies have shown that short- or long-term administration of Ginseng can increase the nonspecific response to various noxious influences, whether physically, chemically, or biologically induced. Even very short-term administration of Ginseng promotes the reestablishment of normal function of the organism. Longer-term use appears to cause numerous physiological changes in the animal or human consuming it, resulting in improved functioning, which becomes more or less permanent.

Ginseng has powerful antifatigue effects, and moderate doses enhance endurance. Ginseng can thus prevent fatigue when consumed prior to exertion. The antifatigue effects are the result of complex metabolic regulatory activities. Primarily, however, it involves significantly improved utilization of glycogen and the reduced accumulation of lactic acid and acetoacetic acid.

The total saponin fragment of Panax Ginseng has been found to have both hypertensive and antihypertensive activity. This has been determined to be due to the coexistence of agonistic and antagonistic saponins in the total saponins. Overall, this coexistence seems to explain the *regulatory* capacity of Ginseng on blood pressure. Russian scientists have reported that Ginseng normalized the level of arterial pressure and that it was clinically effective in the treatment of both hypo- and hypertension, with the exception of severe forms of the latter.

Ginseng both stimulates and inhibits the higher nervous activity. However, the stimulatory action appears to be stronger. A wide range of experiments has proved that the learning ability of laboratory animals is significantly improved when they are fed Ginseng. A double-blind experiment involving Chinese students over a thirty-three-day period showed that Ginseng improved their responses. Ginseng has also been shown to improve the concentration of writers and elderly persons.

The extract of Ginseng has been shown to have mild tranquilizing, analgesic, and muscle-relaxant action. One dominant ginsenoside, Rb_1, has been shown to be tranquilizing, as is the total saponin fraction extracted from Ginseng leaves. The water extract of Ginseng has been shown to have anticonvulsant effects. It can antagonize convulsions caused by cocaine and strychnine, for example. However, at a different dose and with different fractions and different preparation, Ginseng can be stimulating. It has been shown to weaken the effects of strong sedatives. Again, typical water extracts of Ginseng tend to have a normalizing action, thereby helping the body and mind attain optimum nervous activity for whatever action the body and mind are being used for.

The effects on the endocrine system have been studied by hundreds of researchers. Studies have demonstrated that Ginseng is devoid of corticosteroid-like activity. However, it does have a potent influence on the pituitary-adrenal system, and this is one reason why it so profoundly affects the stress reaction in animals and humans. Ginseng is capable of significantly reducing the pathological processes of stress in animals and humans. Ginseng directly influences the pituitary, and probably the hypothalamus, the virtual regulatory centers of the entire hormonal system in higher animals and man. Ginseng appears to influence both the anterior and the posterior pituitary.

Ginseng appears to have profound influence on the gonads of animals. Experiments suggest that Ginseng has no sex-hormone-like action itself, but does appear to have gonadotropin-like action. Many animal experiments have illustrated Ginseng's ability to stimulate sexual behavior. Although Ginseng is widely touted as a sexual tonic, no serious double-blind clinical studies have been conducted to study the validity of this claim. However, castrated rats given Ginseng enter into a mating frenzy. Ovariectomized female rats, given Ginseng in their food, go into sexual mode and are even capable of attracting male rats out of mating season. Human clinical studies have shown that Ginseng is an effective agent for the treatment of impotence and some types of infertility.

Ginseng can promote the lowering of the blood glucose level, but it appears that Asian Ginseng alone cannot prevent or treat diabetes. American Ginseng, it should be noted, has demonstrated a much stronger hypoglycemic effect than Asian Ginseng. Ginsenosides promote the synthesis of cholesterol but decrease the cholesterol in animals with high cholesterol. It has likewise been shown that a peptide in the water extract of Ginseng has antifat-forming action.

Varieties and Grading: It is essential that you know that there are many varieties of Panax Ginseng. No herb in the world comes in more distinct varieties and grades. In selecting a Ginseng root or Ginseng product, the primary considerations are the source and age of the root and the method by which the root was processed. Size, shape, and aroma are also important criteria.

In general, it can be assumed that the wilder, the older, and the richer in flavor and aroma a root is, the better. The source can make all the difference in the world, and proper processing is essential. Authenticity is another important issue, as there are numerous ways to fake high-quality Ginseng, and counterfeiting is rampant in the Ginseng market. Ultimately, however, the only real criterion is efficacy—that is, the bioactivity of the Ginseng and its various components. This is often subjective and may be overt or subtle. In general, Ginseng that grew in the best locations, that is wild or semi-wild, or at least has been grown from superior seed stock, is older than eight years, and is rich in aroma is the kind you are looking for.

Wild Ginseng Root: ★★★★★+ Wild Panax Ginseng grows in deep-shaded forests and hillsides of northeastern China and Korea. It is a shy plant that tends to grow under other plants out of sight of humans. It is never found near stagnant water. Wild Ginseng is much more expensive than cultivated Ginseng. Virtually everybody believes that wild roots are more potent and more chemically balanced than cultivated roots, no matter how carefully the cultivation was handled. However, this is only partly true.

True Wild Ginseng has a long head and is generally smaller than cultivated Ginseng. Wild Ginseng Roots from China can be as old as sixty-five years. Such old roots will have very long heads and will cost thousands of dollars for a root that is less than an ounce in weight. Typical wild roots from China are around fifteen years old. The older the root, the better. These are available at Chinese herb shops.

The best (and most expensive) Wild Ginseng in the world

comes from the Changbai mountain range in northeast China at the border of North Korea. Changbai Mountain is a spectacular volcanic mountain range that is a vast protected-environment preserve. On a recent trip to Changbai Mountain, I was able to stop along the road as we drove and buy thirty-seven genuine wild roots from peasants who were hoping that a Ginseng-loving traveler might stop and buy their treasure. To me this was Ginseng heaven! I was also able to pick wild-growing Schizandra and observe Atractylodes, White Peony, and Acanthopanax (Siberian Ginseng) growing in their natural habitat.

Occasionally, you can find semi-wild white roots. These are roots that were discovered growing wild in the forest, but were then protected and nurtured by the farmer who discovered them. They are usually harvested at a relatively young age of ten years. These, of course, are extremely powerful and match the power of semi-wild red roots. Semi-wild roots, whether white or red, are very similar to true wild roots.

North Korean Red Ginseng: ★★★★★   There are several kinds of premium Red Ginseng grown in Asia. These include South Korean Red, Chinese Shih Chu Red, Korean Semi-Wild Red, and Chinese Emperors' Tribute Red. All of these are absolutely great. North Korea produces premium Red Ginseng. It is not legally available in the United States, but it is widely distributed throughout the rest of the world.

Genuine North Korean Ginseng is considered by many connoisseurs of Ginseng to be the finest cultivated Ginseng in the world. It is very, very powerful. It is also expensive, even in distribution centers such as Hong Kong. It is generally used to provide increased physical power, especially sexual power.

Ginseng can be treated with hot water, then steamed in a closed room, and finally dried, in the process of which it turns a glossy reddish brown. This is known as Red Ginseng. Some preparers add herbs to the steam water, which changes the quality of the Ginseng. For example, though North Korean Ginseng is prepared by a secret process, it is widely assumed that the secret involves adding herbs that increase the potency of the Ginseng. North Korean Ginseng is very *yang* and thus has a hot energy. It is probable that this results from harsh conditions during growth as well as *yang* herbs being added to the steam water.

North Korean Ginseng comes in three grades: Heaven, Earth, and Man. Heaven Grade is the best and the most expensive. It also comes in a variety of sizes: 10, 15, 20, 25, and so on up to 45. The number represents the number of roots that fit into a Chinese "catty." A catty weighs 1.6 U.S. pounds. The description "Heaven Grade 15" Ginseng root means that fifteen Heaven Grade roots make one catty. In other words, the smaller the number, the larger the root. If you're going to buy North Korean Ginseng, only buy Heaven Grade roots and don't bother with a root smaller than a 30. I personally don't bother with roots smaller than a 20. Because larger roots are more potent, they cost more—but it's worth it.

As with all Ginseng, beware of counterfeits. North Korean Ginseng is widely imitated. Far more fake North Korean Ginseng is sold than the real thing, especially in the United States. Real North Korean roots come out of a metal can that has been neatly printed in the factory with red labeling and art on both faces. Counterfeits have a *paper* label wrapped around the can. I never buy a Ginseng root that came out of a tin can with a paper label. They're virtually always counterfeit. Real North Korean Heaven Grade roots are very tasty, while imitations taste much more bland.

South Korean Red Ginseng: ★★★★★   South Korean Ginseng is of very high quality. The Koreans have put enormous effort into trying to make their Ginseng the best in the world.

Recently, more and more experts are saying that South Korean Ginseng is beginning to genuinely rival or even surpass North Korean Ginseng. And South Korean Ginseng is legal in the United States. It is therefore easy to obtain. It is not inexpensive, but it is less expensive than North Korean.

Just like North Korean, South Korean Ginseng is divided into Heaven, Earth, and Man grades and is graded by size. Again, only Heaven Grade is truly great, and larger roots are better. If you buy a South Korean Heaven Grade 15 or 20 root, you will appreciate its obvious potency. South Korean Earth Grade is adequate for maintenance.

Though South Korean Ginseng is widely counterfeited, there is also plenty of the real stuff around. Just check to make sure the root came out of a painted can and not a can wrapped in a paper label.

Chinese Shih Chu Red Ginseng: ★★★★★　　Many people in Asia consider this to be the finest Red Ginseng in the world. Wild seeds are collected and planted in forest beds, where the roots are allowed to develop for a minimum of ten years before harvesting. This technique is only practiced in one place in China, in the Shih Chu Valley in Jilin, near Korea. Supposedly, Shih Chu Valley has the best soil in China for growing Ginseng. Shiu Chu is my favorite Ginseng, next to wild Ginseng. In some cases, it is even better than wild Ginseng, since its energy is more overt.

Shih Chu Ginseng is powerful yet mild. It affects body and mind. It lifts the spirit and sharpens the intellect. It is the perfect Red Ginseng. However, there is a major caveat. Only large Heaven Grade Shih Chu is really good. Shih Chu, like Korean cultivated, comes in the three grades of Heaven, Earth, and Man. Only Heaven Grade is grown from wild seed and allowed to remain in the ground for ten years. Only buy Heaven Grade 16, 20, or 24 roots. Anything smaller is of less potency. And as always, watch out for counterfeits. Real Shih Chu Red

Ginseng comes either in a painted metal can or a similarly designed cardboard box. If it comes in a tin can with a paper label, forget it—it's fake.

This is probably the best Red Ginseng for the majority of people. It is not as *yang* as the Korean reds, which is good for most people, and it is readily available. It is a stunning product and I personally find it to be the perfect tonic herb.

Changbai Mountain Red Ginseng: ★★★★ The finest Ginseng in the world comes from the Changbai Mountain area. Shih Chu Valley is in this area. Throughout the valleys surrounding Changbai Mountain, Ginseng is cultivated on a large scale. Changbai Mountain Ginseng is highly favored by the Chinese and is the most common Ginseng used in China by connoisseurs.

Jilin Commercial-Grade Red Ginseng: ★★★ Ginseng is grown throughout northeastern China. The main provinces where Ginseng grows are Jilin and Heilongjiang, which is north of Jilin. This whole region was formerly known as Manchuria, where it is widely believed that Ginseng originated. Jilin is the main growing region, and most of the world supply of commercial-grade Chinese Ginseng is grown here. In general, the lower the altitude above sea level and the farther from Changbai Mountain, the lower the quality of the Ginseng. Most commercial products use this lower-grade Jilin Ginseng. This is a beneficial herb, but it is not sublime like the premium Ginsengs.

White Ginseng: ★★★ Both South Korea and China export a great deal of White Ginseng. White Ginseng is dried Ginseng that has not been steamed. Either it is peeled and allowed to sun-dry, or it is left to sun-dry with its skin intact. Most White Ginseng has been peeled.

In general, the best roots are prepared as red roots in the

Orient. White roots are milder and more *yin* than red roots. White roots are fine for maintenance.

Standardized Ginseng Products: In an attempt to come to grips with this incredibly wide range of Ginsengs, and the unpredictability of results, the modern nutriceutical industry is attempting to set chemical standards by which Ginseng (and all other herbs) can be judged. This is a wonderful idea, except that I do not believe that there is enough known yet about Ginseng's chemistry to base everything on one chemical standard. For example, I believe it is impossible to say that a 4 percent or 6 percent ginsenoside-standardized Ginseng from one company has any relevance to a 4 percent ginsenoside-standardized extract from another company. Different varieties of Ginseng have different ratios of ginsenosides, which have an entirely different physiological effect. Ginsenosides extracted from Ginseng root are very different from the ginsenosides extracted from stems, rhizomes, or leaves. Different extraction techniques will yield products with vastly different chemical makeups. The resulting effects on one's physiology can vary greatly.

Artificially standardizing Ginseng to a set level of ginsenosides is not an adequate means of judging the quality of the Ginseng you are consuming. Many other factors come into play, besides ginsenoside ratios and quantities. The presence and quantities of other ingredients, such as polysaccharides, germanium, and enzymes, may play a major role in the actual activity of Ginseng. Though standardized Ginseng is consistent and undoubtedly beneficial, I do not believe it is the source of the best Ginseng experience you can obtain. Whole Ginseng extracts from the best sources, properly and caringly prepared, will always provide the best results, even if from batch to batch there may be some deviation of constituents.

The obvious advantage of standardization lies in the ability to do controlled pharmacological and clinical testing. Ginsana™, a major Ginseng brand, conducted such studies on their product between 1980 and the present that have proved their standardized Ginseng extract to be safe and effective. Such clinical trials demonstrated that their product (G115™) improves general physical condition and mental performance, including learning ability, and enhances the nonspecific immunologic functions of the body, thus improving resistance. All in all, seven European clinical studies involving standardized Ginseng (4 percent) were conducted in the 1980s, with results that demonstrated shortening of time to react to auditory and visual stimuli, improved visual and motor coordination, increased alertness, improved grasp of abstract concepts, improved concentration, and increased respiratory quotient. All of this is valuable to most people, and it could easily be said that this makes 4 percent standardized Ginseng an ideal herb for athletes.

All authentic, high-quality Ginseng should at least match, if not far surpass, these results. Does Ginsana provide the *shen* or *qi* that will be available from a wild Ginseng root or from a Shih Chu root? The answer is clearly no. Will it provide the power of a Korean Heaven Grade root? Again the answer is no. Will it be psychically as powerful as a real Heaven Grade Shih Chu root? Not a chance. Is it a good product? Absolutely.

Biotechnology Ginseng: Very strict surrounding conditions, such as soil and climate, are required for cultivating Ginseng. Therefore, the cultivation of Ginseng is very much limited by numerous biological factors. With the advances of modern biological techniques, many scientists in China, Japan, Korea, and Russia have been investigating "tissue cultivation" and "cell cultivation" of Ginseng. They are also investigating cell cultivation in order to produce Ginseng saponins in large quantities sufficient for industrial production. Japan, China, and Russia are all racing to industrialize Ginseng cell culture technology.

Based on over a decade of research, Professor Ding Jiayi of China Pharmaceutical University has developed the cultivation method. Ginseng tissue can be grown from cell culture, without the need to grow in the ground. Professor Ding has painstakingly developed hundreds of strains of Ginseng cell culture, each with its own attributes based on the genome of that particular strain. In general, Professor Ding feels that there are four primary advantages to Ginseng cell culture technology:

1. The quantity of Ginseng saponins can be very high. The crude saponin contents in cultured Ginseng cells can reach 22 percent, in contrast to the 4 percent that is standard for earth-grown, sun-dried Ginseng. However, based on the genome selected and on the nutrients provided to the cell culture, any percentage of saponins desired can be produced on a mass scale and under the complete control of the technicians. Furthermore, Professor Ding is certain that within a few years specific ginsenosides can be generated in predefined ratios, thus creating designer Ginseng which can have clearly defined pharmacological activity based on the amounts and ratios of its constituents.

2. The content of bio-organic germanium (Ge) is controllable. Based on genome selection, certain biotechnological methods, and the amount of inorganic germanium provided as a nutrient, the content of cultured cells can reach 100 parts per million or higher, while earth-cultivated Ginseng contains about 2 ppm. Even wild Ginseng contains only about 5 ppm. Therefore, Ginseng cell culture can become an economical means of producing bio-organic germanium as a specific supplement. Germanium has been linked to the positive functioning of the human immune system and has been recognized in Japan and China as a cancer-preventive agent.

3. The polysaccharide content of Ginseng cell culture can be higher than that of cultivated Ginseng. It has been established that these polysaccharides are responsible for much of Ginseng's immune-potentiating ability. However, normal cultivated Ginseng has a low quantity of polysaccharides. Ginseng cell culture can thus be biotechnologically manipulated to be a stronger immune-potentiating agent.

4. The superoxide dismutase (SOD) activity in the cultured cells is far higher than that of cultivated Ginseng. Dried, earth-grown Ginseng retains almost no SOD activity. However, even after freeze-drying, the SOD activity remains relatively unchanged. This SOD activity makes Ginseng cell culture an ideal ingredient in antiaging cosmetics for topical application, since SOD has been shown to slow the aging of skin.

This is the ultimate in standardization, and this type of technology will probably become common or even prevalent in the next couple of decades as the nutriceutical industry matures. There will always be people who want the real herb, out of the earth. I am one of those. There will be others who prefer standardization. Certainly, for some medical purposes and for use in cosmetics and other products requiring very careful chemistry, standardized extracts will be appropriate, but for pure life enhancement and the development of the Three Treasures, nature will always remain supreme.

Preparation and Utilization: You may cook Ginseng with most other tonic herbs. Slice a root and put it in soup with herbs like Astragalus and Dang Gui. You may also eat small amounts raw. This is a very common practice among true herb connoisseurs. There are so many kinds of Ginseng and so many ways to prepare and consume it that I recommend you ask your Ginseng supplier the best way to use your roots. If you purchase commercially prepared Ginseng products, follow the instructions provided.

There are sources for every type of Ginseng. It is one of the world's most widely used supplements. My company, for example, provides a limited-production extract of the various forms of wild Ginseng (no commercially grown Ginseng included). It is known as Heaven Drops™ Wild Ginseng. Experts from around the world agree that it is in a league by itself.

Contraindications: All authorities agree that Ginseng has a very low acute and chronic toxicity. Over the period of more than two thousand years of continuous use, Ginseng has gained a reputation as being a strong herb, but one that is free of side effects when used moderately and appropriately. Italian researchers have shown that 2,100 mg/kg of Ginseng extract given orally in standard toxicity studies gave no indication of acute toxicity. Long-term, chronic toxicity studies have likewise shown Ginseng to have no negative side effects.

Excessive intake may cause headaches or muscle tension in people of a *yang* constitution. *Yang* varieties of Ginseng should be used with caution and moderately by people with a *yang* constitution or by anyone who is experiencing hot conditions. Ginseng is not to be used by anyone experiencing an acute fever or sore throat.

ACANTHOPANAX (SIBERIAN GINSENG)

Pharmaceutical Name: Radix Acanthopanacis
Treasures: *Qi* and *jing*
Atmospheric Energy: Warm
Taste: Slightly pungent, somewhat bitter and astringent
Organ Associations: Spleen, Lungs, Kidneys, Heart, and Liver
Treasure Rating: ★★★★★

Qualities Attributed to Acanthopanax: The herb widely known as Siberian Ginseng (and as Eleutherococcus) has developed a major reputation as a premier supplement for those who require additional physical strength or who suffer as a result of low resistance to the side effects of extreme exertion. It is especially popular among athletes or physical workers who require substantial sources of adaptive energy and endurance, such as long-distance runners, rock climbers, bicyclists, scuba divers, dancers, tennis players, construction workers, gardeners, and others seeking to enhance physical and mental performance, endurance, and adaptability. It aids in the recovery from hard exercise as well as from extreme mental exertion.

It is now routinely used by people required to engage in high-stress, high energy-demanding activities such as high-altitude flying, long-distance sailing, working in high- or low-temperature environments or in deep water. Acanthopanax has been used by all Russian cosmonauts. The use of the extract of this herb in these endeavors has been reported to increase physical strength, sharpen concentration, improve various parameters of mental power, increase visual acuity, improve color vision, and promote healing power.

Acanthopanax is a very powerful adaptogenic agent. It is among the most famous and important adaptogenic herbs in the world. It helps expand the dimensions of work that one can perform, improving work capacity in both the short and the long term. Athletes and workers all over the world have found that regular consumption of the extract of this herb provides endurance and the capacity to handle heavy workloads with less strain on the body.

Acanthopanax is an extremely safe herb that has been clearly demonstrated to have no negative side effects. It contains no steroids or other dangerous chemical agents. Its benefits are derived from its broad spectrum of eleutherosides, chemical agents that help the nervous and endocrine systems to perform at a higher level. These eleutherosides are saponins, which are very similar to the saponins found in Panax Ginseng, Notoginseng, and Gynostemma.

Acanthopanax increases respiratory power by improving the ability of the body to absorb and efficiently use oxygen. For this reason, Russian cosmonauts use it during space travel. Mountain climbers who scale peaks where oxygen becomes scarce commonly use Acanthopanax to reduce the stress on the body caused by the adverse conditions, and to absorb oxygen more efficiently. For the same reasons, anyone engaged in hard physical activity will benefit from the consumption of Siberian Ginseng. It is a superb athlete's tonic, especially for athletes who rely on respiratory endurance.

Acanthopanax helps *regulate* functions so that optimum physiological *efficiency* is achieved. Used regularly, the energy of the whole body will increase. This herb has been shown to reduce the activation of the adrenal cortex in response to stress, which means that it helps to prevent excessive stress reactions, which can damage other components of the endocrine and nervous systems and result in exhaustion. In clinical trials in which Acanthopanax was administered to healthy human subjects, results showed that Acanthopanax increases the ability to withstand a wide range of adverse physical and mental conditions, such as intense exercise, increase in workload, noise, heat, motion, and decompression. It was also shown in the same studies to improve athletic performance and the quality of work under stressful conditions. The herb is very widely used to prevent altitude sickness, a disorder associated with oxygen deficiency.

Besides being characterized as a tonic herb, Acanthopanax is also regarded as a mild but significant stimulant. This stimulating action refers to the pharmacological ability of Acanthopanax to increase the work capacity of a person after a single dose of the preparation. This is in some contrast to its tonic action, which refers to its ability to increase work capacity after prolonged or continuous consumption of the herb. Work capacity is increased as a result of taking a tonic, not just during the time period when the substance is being used, but for a sustained period of time afterward. Thus Acanthopanax has the rare ability to increase both immediate energy and long-term energy and is therefore known as a stimulating tonic. It increases the general tone of the body while adjusting and normalizing arterial blood pressure and blood sugar levels. It does not possess the negative side effects, depressing qualities, or addictive potential of most other pharmacological and biological stimulants such as coffee, guarana, amphetamines, and cocaine. It is the safest and healthiest known stimulant.

Acanthopanax has been shown to improve mental alertness and work output. Numerous studies have demonstrated that Acanthopanax has the ability to enhance sensorial perception, improving visual acuity and night vision and heightening auditory awareness, all while protecting the eyes and hearing apparatus from damage due to excess stimulation.

In addition, considerable research and clinical evidence have demonstrated that Acanthopanax is a powerful immune modulator. It helps to build resistance to infectious disease and can prevent autoimmune reactions. Studies have shown that Acanthopanax is especially useful in reducing the incidence of influenza in groups of people who consume it regularly.

The extract of Acanthopanax is widely used clinically in Asia. It is broadly used as an adjunct in the treatment of chronic diseases, where numerous reports indicate that the herb increases physical strength of patients, especially those who have undergone surgery, severe acute illness, and exhaustion. The root extract is commonly used clinically to relieve the symptoms and pain due to rheumatic arthritis. The herb is also used clinically in China during the treatment of diabetes mellitus. Acanthopanax has been shown to promote antibody formation and to protect the immune system, in particular to prevent leukopenia (depressed white blood cell count) due to various cytotoxins.

The remarkable normalizing ability of Acanthopanax was again demonstrated when it was shown to regulate the red and white blood cells. After profuse bleeding, Acanthopanax promotes the recovery of hemoglobin and stimulates antibody production. Similarly, Acanthopanax normalized blood pressure in laboratory animals, where the blood pressure was high or low to start with. This regulatory effect of Acanthopanax has been observed clinically in humans. Therefore, Acanthopanax is used clinically in China, Korea, Russia, and Japan to regulate blood pressure. Blood pressure in either hypertensive or hypotensive patients generally normalizes after oral administration of Acanthopanax, according to numerous clinical reports.

It has been demonstrated that Acanthopanax has anabolic action which can result in an increase in lean body weight. Acanthopanax, however, differs from the steroid anabolic hormones. It does not have a masculinizing effect.

Acanthopanax has also been demonstrated to be a remarkably safe substance. No abnormalities resulted from administration of Acanthopanax to mice at 350 g/kg, a very high dosage. When mice were given doses 220 times the clinical dose, they showed no abnormalities after seven days. The animals were able to tolerate administration of the herb extract throughout their life spans without toxic reactions. In fact, continuous treatment for six months prolonged their average life span and did not adversely affect ensuing offspring.

All this adds up to one of the most useful and powerful health supplements known to mankind. In an era when work-loads are intense, stress is ubiquitous, and competition is the name of the game, Acanthopanax is the perfect adaptogenic substance to make part of your daily regimen. Those who use high-quality Acanthopanax quickly discover that it is one of the great tools in nature's herbal arsenal. It provides an abundance of both quick and long-term energy that results in an improved ability to handle stress and further results in the improvement of one's capacities, both physical and mental.

Varieties and Grading: There is considerable confusion in the world market as to how to determine true Siberian Ginseng. True Acanthopanax comes from either Russian Siberia or the northernmost province of China, Heilongjiang, which is a frigid area adjacent to Russian Siberia. The herb itself is the woody root of the aboveground shrub. It is very difficult to find raw Acanthopanax root in herb stores in America. Because of its woody nature, it takes a large quantity of the root to yield even a small amount of extract. Generally, it takes fifty pounds of Acanthopanax root to produce one pound of finished extract powder. For this reason, it is generally found only as a finished product in extract form. Most Acanthopanax is processed in China and sold in America either as concentrated powder in capsules and pills or as liquid concentrates. The best extracts are dark in color and are strongly bitter in flavor.

Do not get this herb confused with *Acanthopanax gracilistylus* (Chinese: *wu jia pi*), which is the root bark of a related species used specifically in Chinese herbalism to treat rheumatism, but which does not have the tonic qualities of *Acanthopanax senticosus*, true Siberian Ginseng. This medicinal Acanthopanax is the herb sold at Chinese herb shops in

Chinatowns throughout America. You will not find Siberian Ginseng sold in bulk in most Chinese herb shops.

Preparation and Utilization: Since in virtually all cases this product is sold as an extracted powder or elixir, simply follow instructions on the product you purchase. The liquid extract may be added to teas and combined with other tonic herbs.

Contraindications: None.

AMERICAN GINSENG ROOT

Pharmaceutical Name: Radix Panax Quinquefolium
Treasures: *Yin* and *qi*
Atmospheric Energy: Cool
Taste: Sweet and slightly bitter
Organ Associations: Lungs, Spleen, and Stomach
Treasure Rating: ★★★★★

Qualities Attributed to the Root: American Ginseng is not the same herb as Asian Ginseng. Though it is used in much the same way and with many of the same goals in mind, American Ginseng is different in its actions from the Asian varieties. American Ginseng is an adaptogenic and a *qi* tonic. It thus provides energy, adaptability, and heightened alertness. It is especially appreciated for its endurance-increasing capacity.

However, American Ginseng is a *yin* tonic and is cool in nature. This is in contrast to Asian Ginseng, which is a *yang* tonic and is generally warm, or even hot, in nature. American Ginseng is useful for people who are hot but wish to take Ginseng. In other words, people who have lots of energy, high metabolisms, are aggressive, have high blood pressure, or have ruddy complexions can take American Ginseng without fear of overheating. In fact, taking the American Ginseng will help to balance out the system and can correct overheating problems, especially when the excess heat is in the lungs and stomach. American Ginseng is often used in China to tonify the lungs of people who have dry coughs due to smog, smoking, or other causes. It is said to moisten and cool the lungs.

American Ginseng is also popular among people who live in warmer climates. Since it is a cooling herb and replenishes fluids, it is especially beneficial during hot weather. American Ginseng is more widely used in southern China than Chinese Ginseng is. However, in the north where the winters are cold,

Chinese Ginseng is still favored. Many people now prefer a blend of American and Asian Ginsengs, with a shift in balance as the seasons turn, using more American Ginseng in the warm months and more Asian Ginseng in the cold months.

American Ginseng is highly regarded for its ability to promote the secretion of body fluids. It is also considered to be especially strengthening to new mothers.

Grades and Varieties: Though Asian varieties of Ginseng are still highly regarded in China, American Ginseng is currently the rage, especially wild American, and probably will remain so, as long as the prices for American Ginseng remain lower than the prices for premium Chinese and Korean Ginsengs. American wild Ginseng is much more readily available at much more favorable prices. Wild American Ginseng is not cheap by any stretch of the imagination, but it is a bargain compared to genuine Chinese wild roots.

Wild American Ginseng grows in many places in North America, from as far south as Missouri to the Hudson Bay. The best wild American Ginseng grows in upstate New York, in the Catskill Mountains and on up into Canada. Wild Ginseng from Wisconsin can be excellent, but that from Pennsylvania, Kentucky, and farther south is considered to be much less potent. As with Asian Ginseng, older roots from more isolated regions are more valuable. Roots that are twenty years old or older are quite expensive. The deeper and tighter the striation on the roots, the harder the Ginseng had to work to survive. Therefore, highly striated Ginseng is better than less deeply striated specimens. I tend to buy only Ginseng that still has its head attached. In that way I can tell if it is a truly old root. The longer the head and the more nodes on the head, the older the root. Roots over twenty years old are considered premium.

Cultivated American Ginseng is a fine *yin* tonic but does not have the potency of *wild* American Ginseng Roots or even a number of other premium *yin* tonics such as Chinese wild Asparagus Root. A very old, very wild American Ginseng Root from the Catskills or Canada is a great thing. Everyone needs *yin*, so American Ginseng is a great herb for everyone, and premium wild roots are a treasure.

Preparation and Utilization: Use as you would use Panax or Siberian Ginseng for energy. American Ginseng comes in a multitude of varieties. Raw roots can be cooked with other herbs, either *yin* tonics or *yang* tonics as desired. If you like, combine it with other varieties of Ginseng to create a balanced Ginseng blend that suits your constitution and condition. Fresh roots are sometimes available from herb shops in the fall for a short period of time. One or two fresh roots may be placed in a bottle of fine alcohol (32 percent or higher) and extracted for a month or longer before consuming one ounce per day, or less often if desired, as a tonic.

Contraindications: None.

ASTRAGALUS ROOT

Pharmaceutical Name: Radix Astragalus
Treasures: *Qi* and Blood
Atmospheric Energy: Warm
Taste: Sweet
Organ Associations: Spleen and Lungs
Treasure Rating: ★★★★★

Qualities Attributed to the Root: Astragalus ranks as one of the most potent health tonics in the world. For over two thousand years, it has been one of the most popular tonic herbs used in the Orient, and remains so.

Astragalus is said to strengthen the primary energy of the body and all metabolic, respiratory, and eliminative functions. As an energizer, Astragalus is famed for its strengthening effects, in particular to the musculature. It is therefore beneficial to those who tend to be physically active and require abundant physical energy. In China, Astragalus is sometimes considered superior to Ginseng as an energizer for younger people. Astragalus is used to strengthen the legs and arms and is commonly used by people who work outdoors, especially in the cold, because of its strengthening and warming nature.

Astragalus is also said to have an effect on the "surface" of the body—it tonifies the "protective *qi*," known as *wei qi* in Chinese. This protective *qi* is a special kind of energy that circulates just under the skin and in the muscle. Protective *qi* is a *yang* energy.

Protective *qi* circulates in the subcutaneous tissues, providing suppleness to the flesh and adaptive energy to the skin. This function is essential to life. This adaptive energy at the surface of the body is our first line of defense against the offensive forces of nature. Astragalus helps the body generate an abundance of free-flowing protective *qi*, thus fortifying the defense energy of the body. Consistent consumption of Astragalus is thus used to protect the body and has traditionally been called the Great Protector.

An important effect of Astragalus is to fortify the "upright *qi*." Upright *qi* is the energy allocated by the body to maintain upright posture and to maintain the position of the organs in their battle with gravity. As one gets older, or if one experiences chronic fatigue or exhaustion, or during illness, this upright *qi* is easily depleted, resulting in the sinking, or prolapse, of organs. This can happen almost anywhere in the body, but it is common in the abdominal and pelvic cavities, where organs tend to sink. Astragalus provides an abundance of this upright *qi*. Thus Astragalus is used for such conditions as hernias and prolapse of the uterus and stomach as well as the inability to stand straight due to fatigue.

Astragalus enhances the function of the skin to eliminate toxins. It is commonly used to help sores in the skin to come to a head and suppurate and thus to heal more quickly and effectively. Astragalus is used by Chinese doctors to help slow-healing sores and wounds heal more quickly. All this activity is related to the protective *qi* that is circulating in the skin, which also improves blood circulation according to the rule of "*qi* leads blood."

Astragalus has a mild diuretic action and helps to relieve excessive sweating. It is helpful in treating loose stools, chronic diarrhea, and chronic or recurring colds. If a cold lasts too long, it can cause a general fatigue syndrome that can itself become chronic. Astragalus is useful for people who can't shake a cold, and Astragalus can replace the *qi* necessary to regain full strength. In China, there are patent medicines consisting solely or primarily of Astragalus that are specifically targeted at treating low-grade chronic colds.

Astragalus is quite effective as a blood tonic when combined with major blood tonic herbs such as Dang Gui.

Astragalus extracts have been proved to have potent immunomodulating effects in both animals and humans. Water extracts of Astragalus enhance macrophage activity and reduce the activity of suppresser T cells. The herbal extract increases natural killer-cell cytotoxicity, helps antibody response, and increases helper-cell activity. Studies conducted at the M. D. Anderson Cancer Research Center at the University of Houston, the world's largest cancer research institute, demonstrated that Astragalus improves the immune response in humans undergoing radiation and chemotherapy as a treatment of cancer. The FDA, however, has not approved the use of Astragalus for this purpose, although it is approved for exactly that purpose in many other countries. It tends to protect the white cells from leukopenia (destruction of white blood cells due to the chemotherapy or radiation) and maintains the healthy activity of these immune cells. Patients taking Astragalus during such treatment tend to have far fewer side effects and to recover at a higher and faster rate.

The primary active constituents of Astragalus, the triterpene glycosides, are saponins similar to the saponins in Ginseng and Gynostemma, though all of the Astragalus saponins have their own chemical identities. There are over thirty such saponins in *Astragalus membranaceus*, for example, of which many are unique to that species. The "total Astragaloside" fraction of Astragalus is an extremely potent health agent. Studies have demonstrated that the "total Astragaloside" fraction has bipolar, biphasic, double-direction activity. It is an extremely potent immune modulator, capable of building the immune response while suppressing excessive immune activity, as occurs in autoimmune conditions (including allergies and arthritis). In addition, the total Astragaloside fraction has a similarly potent antioxidant activity, hundreds of times stronger than vitamin E and stronger than that of Grape Seed extract, *Ginkgo biloba*, and Pine Bark extract. New technology allows this total Astragaloside fraction to be extracted. The new high-potency Astragalus extract, known as TA-70, is without doubt among the most potent health tonic agents in the world today.

The polysaccharides found in Astragalus are also extremely potent immune enhancers. However, these polysaccharides have been shown to be poorly absorbed in the intestines and therefore have a low bioavailability. Pharmacological studies have shown that injected polysaccharides and injected Astragalus glycosides have approximately equivalent potency relating to the immune system, but the glycoside component is five times more potent than the polysaccharides when consumed orally.

Both polysaccharide and saponin fractions have shown liver-protective action. Of the two, the liver-protective action of the saponin fraction is more powerful due to higher bioavailability.

An interesting new area of research on Astragalus concerns its potential as a male fertility agent. Astragalus has been shown to stimulate sperm motility.

Varieties and Grading: Astragalus is one of the premium Chinese tonic herbs and has been a staple of traditional Chinese herbalism for three thousand years. Thus many varieties are available at any Chinese herb shop, ranging in price from very inexpensive to relatively expensive—a few dollars per pound up to around sixty dollars a pound for the best sliced Astragalus. The Astragalus we get in America has been sliced and pressed, which make it appear bigger than it actually was in the ground and also makes it easier to cook or otherwise extract.

If you compare the best Astragalus with the low-end material, you will note a fineness to the quality of the better root slices. Slices that are supple and pliable, which usually indicates that the herb is fresher and was more carefully prepared, are more desirable than dry, brittle slices. High-quality Astragalus has an inner core that is distinctly earthy-yellow. Lesser grades are characterized by a nondistinct whitish-beige core and rough texture. Some unscrupulous suppliers actually dye this inside core yellow. The yellow core is essential, but make sure it is natural (it won't turn a wet tissue artificially yellow).

Good-quality Astragalus has a sweet flavor that is pleasant when cooked in tea. Lower-grade Astragalus is bland and has a starchy taste, or is tasteless.

My recommendation: Buy middle- or high-priced Astragalus. Herb shops don't sell the poor-quality stuff for high prices because too many people are experts in Astragalus. At least buy a middle grade, and preferably buy the best—you'll notice the difference.

Preparation and Utilization: Astragalus may be added to almost any tonic formulation designed to strengthen the entire body. It is superb for young or older people, male or female. It can be the main ingredient or a secondary ingredient. My recommendation here is to consume Astragalus every day, to some degree or another.

Contraindications: Being in the legume family, Astragalus tends to produce flatulence in those who are prone to this distressing symptom when they eat legumes such as peas. If this is the case, use less and try adding herbs like cardamom to the tea. It should not be used during the acute phase of the flu but is highly recommended during the convalescing stage.

DEER ANTLER

Pharmaceutical Name: Cornu Cervi Pantotrichum

Treasures: *Jing* (*yin* and *yang*), *qi* (especially Blood), and *shen*

Atmospheric Energy: Warm

Taste: Sweet and salty

Organ Associations: Liver and Kidneys

Treasure Rating: ★★★★★

Qualities Attributed to Deer Antler: Deer Antler is the most precious and the most potent of the substances that fortify the *yang* energy of the Kidneys, *yang jing*. It is widely used in Asia to strengthen adrenal, reproductive, and brain functions. It is universally believed in the Orient to build sexual strength and to increase virility and fertility. Deer Antler is available in the Asian market in a wide variety of expensive elixirs and combinations that are essentially claimed to be aphrodisiac and antiaging. In the eminently regarded tenth-century Daoist manual on health and sexual conduct, *The Essence of Medical Prescriptions*, it is said that "there is nothing better than deer antler to cause a man to be robust and unaffected by age, not to tire in the bedroom, and not to deteriorate either in energy or in facial coloration."

Like all *yang* herbs, Deer Antler is used to strengthen the back, knees, and waist, but Deer Antler is considered to be the most powerful such agent and is usually the main herb in any formula in which it is included. It is also widely used to improve mental power.

Deer Antler has always been used to help build blood and improve circulation, and modern research has supported its reputation as a Heart tonic. Particularly the alcohol extract of Deer Antler, known as pantocrin, is consumed for this purpose. Deer Antler is tonic to the marrow, which produces blood. Marrow tends to degenerate as we age, and Deer Antler is believed to slow down or reverse this process. This is a major aspect of Deer Antler's youth-preserving ability.

Research indicates that moderate doses of pantocrin (primarily the alcohol extract of Deer Antler) benefit cardiovascular function by helping to regulate heart rhythm and by improving circulation in people with chronic poor circulation.

Deer Antler is mainly used as a rejuvenating agent. Short-term use is believed to quickly build strength and power, while consistent long-term use is believed to rebuild deep life force, preserve youthfulness or even reverse aging, and enhance longevity.

Deer Antler is a rare type of organ in the higher animal kingdom. It is one of the few complex organ structures that regenerate in an annual rhythm, and it will also regenerate if cut or broken off. This regenerative power is what has most intrigued scientists in recent years, just as it has the Asian people through the ages.

Studies conducted in Europe indicate that the ability to regenerate is due to the rich supply of substances known as ectosaponins. This complex chemical agent is found more abundantly in lower animals, in which the ectosaponins cause a wide variety of tissue to regenerate. The ectosaponin in Deer Antler is very similar to ectosaponins found at the tail bases of many lizards, such as the gecko, and in the legs of starfish. Just as in the case of Deer Antler, if the tail is broken off a gecko or similar lizard or the legs broken off a starfish, these appendages regrow—bone, nerves, blood vessels, flesh and all. The ectosaponins extracted from Deer Antler as well as from gecko and starfish have shown remarkable regenerative effects on all types of tissue, including nerve tissue, which generally does not regenerate well.

Numerous studies done in China, Japan, and Korea have shown that Deer Antler increases work capacity, decreases muscular and mental fatigue, and improves sleep and appetite. Deer Antler has been shown to increase the oxygen uptake of the brain, liver, and kidneys in laboratory animals. It also significantly increased red and white blood cell production in laboratory animals, with the effects increasing as dose was increased.

Grades and Varieties: There are many grades, cuts, and qualities of Deer Antler—and there are some counterfeits. Larger antlers are produced by deer who are more sexual, and this Deer Antler is more potent. Size alone, however, will tell you little about quality.

Deer Antler can have a number of origins. High-quality Deer Antler entering the American market may originate in China, Russia, Mongolia, or New Zealand. None originates in the Americas. Deer antlers are cut off living deer early each summer. The deer are not killed or really harmed. The deer herds are carefully protected and maintained. They are worth much more alive and healthy than sick or dead.

Deer Antler is available in a very wide range of presentations. Most deer Antler is sold in Chinese herb shops sliced into thin, wafer-thick pieces for easy cooking, extraction, or grinding. This practice is risky to the consumer who does not know much about Deer Antler because it is difficult to know exactly what you are getting unless you have developed an acute eye for it (or unless you trust the herbalist selling it).

There are some really superb concentrated liquid Deer Antler extracts on the market. For most people, these are the best bet. They contain all the active constituents and are a very good value even though they have a fairly high price tag. Good extracts are thick and strong-tasting.

Don't buy cheap Deer Antler—there is no such thing. Bargain-basement antler is probably counterfeit or very old. It may be from a type of deer that is considered to be of little health value, or it may not be from a deer at all. Deer Antler is very valuable—and expensive—so enter the purchasing process with the attitude that you are going to get something really special. The "tips" are the most potent and expensive part of the antler, followed by what are known as "middles."

Preparation and Utilization: Deer Antler can be boiled or even consumed as raw ground powder. A half an ounce, or even a full ounce, in a half gallon of water, brewed with various tonic herbs that suit your constitution, current health condition and needs, is an excellent idea several times a year, if not more often. Mix with Ginseng, Rehmannia, Cordyceps, Ganoderma, et cetera. Make it the king herb, or at least the co-king with Ginseng or Ganoderma.

You can also extract Deer Antler in alcohol. Put several ounces of Deer Antler into a half gallon of 40 percent or stronger alcohol, along with other tonic herbs, and allow to extract for six weeks or longer. You may drink one ounce a night as a superb tonic.

Contraindications: Not to be used during the acute stage of the flu or a cold, or when experiencing acute fever.

CORDYCEPS

Pharmaceutical Name: Cordyceps
Treasures: *Yin jing, yang jing,* and *qi*
Atmospheric Energy: Warm
Taste: Sweet
Organ Associations: Kidneys and Lungs
Treasure Rating: ★★★★★

Qualities Attributed to the Fungus: Cordyceps is one of the absolute superstars of the Chinese tonic herbal system. It is an extremely effective and powerful life-enhancing agent, ranking right up there with Ginseng, Ganoderma, and Deer Antler. Because it is rare, potent, and highly treasured, like Deer Antler, it is very expensive. It is the main ingredient in a number of elite elixirs and tonic formulations.

Cordyceps is used to strengthen the body and mind at a fundamental level. It is said to be able to increase the "primary motive force for life activities." Because it contains both *yin* and *yang*, it can be used by anyone safely and over a long period of time. It replenishes *yin jing*, restoring the deep energy expended as a result of excessive exertion, adapting to stress, or aging. Cordyceps is thus one of the primary herbal substances used in tonic herbalism as an antiaging agent and for the purposes of rejuvenation.

Cordyceps is very widely used to strengthen the primal Kidney functions, which include sexual functions, brainpower, structural integrity, and healing ability. It is a very powerful *yang* tonic. As a sexual tonic, Cordyceps is considered to be one of the best. It is not as quick-acting as the best of the *yang* tonics like Deer Antler, Epimedium, and Sea Dragon, but it has a profound long-term strengthening capacity. It is commonly used for impotence, sexual malaise, frigidity, and infertility.

Consistent use of Cordyceps helps to strengthen the skeletal structure, specifically the lower back region, the knees, and the ankles. It is used for backache due to injury, fatigue, stress, or simple aging.

Cordyceps is also a major Lung tonic. It can be used to strengthen respiratory power in those who require extra energy in order to perform physical work (e.g., labor, sports, or exercise), or it can be used by those who suffer from deficiency of Lung power. It is especially beneficial to those who suffer chronic lung weakness with cough, wheezing, or shortness of breath.

Cordyceps is considered in Asia to be a powerful athletes' tonic. It has no steroidal constituents yet greatly improves performance and muscle-building capability.

Cordyceps is highly regarded in China as a tonic for those who are recovering from an illness or an operation, or after giving birth. In these cases, the Cordyceps helps the patient recover physical power, improves appetite, and protects the body from infection. When blended with other tonics such as Ginseng, Ganoderma, Lycium, or Astragalus, Cordyceps' power is increased, as the synergy of the various herbs results in an even more powerful tonic.

Many studies now indicate that Cordyceps can help the body resist a wide range of pathogenic bacteria, fungi, and viruses. Cordyceps is used in Asia to help treat fungus and yeast infections, and intensive research is being conducted at dozens of institutions in China and Japan relating to the potential of Cordyceps to treat cancer and HIV infection. Researchers in Japan and China have isolated a number of polysaccharides in Cordyceps that strengthen the immune system, and at least one, CO-1, has been shown to have strong antitumor activity. Maintaining the immune system is one of the mechanisms that can slow down aging and prevent both degenerative and acquired diseases.

Other studies have shown that Cordyceps can have a benefit in the vascular system as well. Cordyceps improves the function of the microcirculation and improves efficiency at the capillary level. Cordyceps has been shown to help regulate blood pressure and strengthen heart muscle.

Varieties and Grading: Cordyceps is one of the most rare and expensive herbs in Chinese tonic herbalism. It is a mushroom. The mushroom grows on the head of a caterpillar. The caterpillar is completely consumed by the mushroom but retains its shape. Therefore, it appears just like a dried caterpillar. In fact, however it is now 100 percent vegetarian fungal material.

It is primarily collected wild in the high mountainous regions of Tibet and on the high peaks of China. It can also be grown in a semi-wild manner, but this Cordyceps will be of lower quality (it is still very good). A rule of thumb—low-cost Cordyceps is not wild. The wild Cordyceps will always be the most expensive. In buying Cordyceps, you have to trust your herbalist. Fortunately, all Cordyceps is good—it's just that some is better than others. High-grade Cordyceps is light brown in color and neat. Cordyceps possesses a rich and not unpleasant flavor.

Wild Cordyceps from Tibet is the best Cordyceps in the world. The very best Cordyceps, the kind the emperor or empress would want, is called Imperial Cordyceps. It is graded according to size, the larger the better.

The difference between Tibetan Cordyceps and wild Chinese Cordyceps is actually not that significant. However, there *is* a big difference between wild and cultivated Cordyceps. They look alike, but studies have shown that wild Cordyceps is richer in certain components and that the proportions of components is different, which probably makes a difference in the activity. However, cultivated Cordyceps is still a premium tonic herb, and if this is what you can find, it's still great (★★★★). The Cordyceps most commonly found in Chinese herb stores is cultivated. It comes in neat packages. Wild Cordyceps from

China is readily available if you ask for it. Tibetan, however, is rare and precious.

In the last several years, it has become possible to grow a number of fungi by "fermentation" technology. The biomass is literally grown in large tanks, and in just a matter of days a large quantity can be produced. The technology has now become highly advanced and is making previously rare herbs like Cordyceps and Ganoderma much more accessible. Many studies indicate that the chemical nature of this biotechnology Cordyceps is almost identical to that of the wild variety, and pharmacological and clinical studies seem to confirm this. The Cordyceps contained in most commercial products is produced by this technology.

A benefit of growing Cordyceps by fermentation technology is that it is far less expensive to grow a ton of Cordyceps in a tank in just a matter of days than it is to collect a ton of wild Cordyceps off the cliffs of a Tibetan or Chinese peak. Moreover, collecting wild Cordyceps is dangerous work, resulting in injuries every year as collectors fall off cliffs trying to collect this valuable treasure. Until now, few people in the West had even heard of Cordyceps because of its rarity. In the next decade, as a result of the new fermentation technology, Cordyceps will become known throughout the world.

There is one more advantage, at least by some people's standards, to the new fermentation Cordyceps. There's no caterpillar! Wild Cordyceps, by weight, is mostly caterpillar, and Americans generally don't eat caterpillars. Certainly, even if wild Cordyceps were readily available, most Americans would be turned off by the sight of what appears to be a caterpillar (most people call it a worm) or even just the thought of it. Frankly, it doesn't matter at all, since in reality there is not a trace of the caterpillar left. The entire thing has become a mushroom. Only the shape of the caterpillar remains. Still, it may be of interest to some that the fermentation process does not use animal nutrients, and the result is a 100 percent pure vegetarian health product.

Preparation and Utilization: Combine with other premium herbs to create amazing elixirs. Use anywhere from a few grams up to half an ounce, according to your needs and your budget. Cordyceps is very safe and may be used in large quantities if you are wealthy.

Contraindications: Not to be used when experiencing a fever.

GYNOSTEMMA

Pharmaceutical Name: Herba Gynostemma
Treasures: *Jing, qi,* and *shen*
Atmospheric Energy: Slightly cool
Taste: Sweet and slightly bitter
Organ Associations: Spleen, Lungs, Kidneys, Liver, and Heart
Treasure Rating: ★★★★★

Qualities Attributed to the Herb: Gynostemma is popularly believed in Asia to be an antiaging, longevity herb. Gynostemma is generally reinforcing to overall health and has a strong antifatigue effect. It is also used as a virtual "cure-all." Gynostemma is a major adaptogenic herb, in the same league as Panax Ginseng, Acanthopanax (Siberian Ginseng), Ganoderma, Schizandra, and Astragalus.

It was reported in 1972 that Gynostemma was used in southern China to successfully treat senile chronic bronchitis. This drew the attention of researchers from around the world, and Japanese researchers in particular took note. Japanese investigators soon visited China to study the situation. They found that the reports were accurate. Further investigation indicated that the southern Chinese people used Gynostemma to treat not only chronic bronchitis but a wide variety of other problems and health conditions, and even more important, they used it as a longevity herb. It was discovered by the Japanese researchers that many Chinese octogenarians drank Gynostemma daily. This led the Japanese to do research into the constituents and pharmacology of Gynostemma, which in turn led to the confirmation that the herb possesses an incredibly broad range of phytochemicals and health benefits.

Since the 1980s, Japanese and Chinese researchers have mounted a large-scale investigation of the plant and its saponins. Japanese botanists developed an especially sweet variety of Gynostemma. The Japanese herb industry sent these seeds to China for mass cultivation, and by the late 1980s, the majority of cultivated Gynostemma in China was of this sweet variety. In recent years, numerous products have been developed in both Japan and China. The Japanese have patented dozens of products using Gynostemma and its active constituents. Gynostemma has become one of the most popular tonic herbs in Asia.

In China, Gynostemma is widely believed to have the following health benefits: to slow down aging and prevent feebleness at all ages, and in particular to prevent senility; to reduce fatigue and increase vigor; to reduce oxygen deficiency at high altitudes; to improve digestion; to strengthen the mind; to improve sex functions; to help calm the nerves; and to ease pain.

The ultimate greatness of Gynostemma lies in its broad-spectrum adaptogenic quality. It has double-direction activity in many areas. It has the ability to bring balance to the body under a wide range of stressful circumstances. Constant consumption of Gynostemma tends to have a highly protective quality because it strengthens the adaptive capacity of the person at every level of life. The chemical constituents responsible for the adaptogenic characteristic of Gynostemma are saponins called gypenosides.

Gynostemma contains more than eighty different gypenosides. This is the broadest range of saponins in one plant in nature. Ginseng has about thirty-six saponins (ginsenosides) and Astragalus has about thirty-two (astragalosides). The gypenosides are very similar to the ginsenosides of Ginseng and to the eleutherosides of Acanthopanax (Siberian Ginseng). In fact, four of Gynostemma's saponins are precisely the same chemical structure as the saponins found in Ginseng, and eleven more are almost identical. The similarities are so close and so extensive that Gynostemma is now called Southern Ginseng. To the local people who grow it and consume it, it is simply called Magical Grass.

Gynostemma contains many amino acids, vitamins, and minerals that are healthful to the human body, including selenium, magnesium, zinc, calcium, iron, potassium, manganese, and phosphorus.

Japanese studies have indicated that Gynostemma has a double-direction, regulating, adaptogenic influence on the central nervous system. It is calming when one is overexcited and stimulating when one is depressed. Japanese studies have shown that Gynostemma is clinically useful in a number of mental and neurological conditions, including simple depression, anxiety, and schizophrenia.

Though Gynostemma is regarded as a tonic herb, it is also perceived by many Asian people to be a cure-all. In China, Gynostemma is being used to treat inflammation, stop cough, remove mucus, treat chronic bronchitis, and much more in actual clinical practice.

Gynostemma has developed an enormous reputation in Asia as a major aid in weight control programs. It has a double-direction activity with regard to weight. It will help reduce weight in overweight people and can help athletes, bodybuilders, or excessively slim people gain weight. As a diet herb, it helps by accelerating the body's metabolism. It also helps adjust blood sugar and reduce blood fat. Adjusting blood sugar and blood fat are critical steps in attaining healthy metabolic function, whether one wants to lose or gain weight. Gynostemma has been shown to have profound effects in reducing simple obesity. Japanese and Chinese studies indicate that Gynostemma lowers low-density lipoprotein (LDL—"bad" cholesterol) while increasing high-density lipoprotein (HDL—"good" cholesterol). Its total efficacious rate has reached 94.8 percent after pharmaceutical and clinical application. It also exerts the effects of fat metabolism accommodation, lipoid peroxide depression, and fat sediment reduction in the blood vessels. Therefore, it is efficacious against arteriosclerosis, coronary heart disease, and simple obesity, providing that such treatment is conducted under the supervision of a qualified primary health care provider.

It has been found that athletes who consume Gynostemma put on more lean muscle than those who do not, probably due to the high saponin content of Gynostemma. Athletes find that their appetites improve and that assimilation is much more efficient.

Although Gynostemma is not a laxative, it will help in the case of constipation and helps maintain healthy bowel movements in people with no problem. It acts as a scavenger in the stomach and intestines, ridding the body of toxins, microbes, and waste that otherwise may become lodged in the intestines. All of these benefits are important to people who are trying to lose or gain weight.

Gynostemma is strengthening to the human immune system. It is used to potentiate immune response and to treat a wide variety of infectious conditions.

Studies into the anticancer activity of Gynostemma have shown a significant (20–80 percent) inhibition rate on a wide range of cancer cells. Intensive studies are now being conducted into both its anticancer activity and its potential as an immune protection/prophylactic agent for HIV-infected individuals. There is recent research indicating that Gynostemma likely prevents cells from becoming cancerous.

Recent medical literature, in both China and Japan, is full of reports on the consistent clinical effectiveness of Gynostemma for an incredibly wide range of health problems, including high blood pressure, coronary heart disease, migraines, diabetes, insomnia, the common cold, gum inflammation, gastric ulcers, gastritis, hemorrhoids, arthritis, rheumatism, neuralgia, hypertrophy of the prostate, chronic pneumonia, acne, warts, gout, various allergies, asthma, otitis media, chronic headaches, and premature graying or loss of hair.

Gynostemma pentaphyllum helps alleviate the side effects induced by steroid drugs.

Varieties and Grading: Growing widely throughout Asia, *Gynostemma pentaphyllum* is a perennial, creeping herb. The content of the total saponins can be used as a main standard in the determination of quality.

Gynostemma, as it comes to market, comes in several grades. The best grows wild in pristine mountain areas of southeastern China, away from cities and industrial pollution. Wild Gynostemma is much more rare than the commercially grown product. Wild Gynostemma is quite bitter, but with a sweet aftertaste. It is hardly ever used in beverages because of its strong bitter flavor. However, connoisseurs appreciate it because of its profound efficacy. Wild Gynostemma contains approximately 15 percent gypenosides, which is quite high. A few exclusive sources sell wild Gynostemma as tea or in capsules.

Commercially farmed Gynostemma is much sweeter than the wild variety. The Japanese developed a strain of Gynostemma known as Sweet Gynostemma. This Sweet Gynostemma is now the primary variety of Gynostemma grown commercially in China and is consumed throughout Asia. It has a light, pleasant flavor with a slightly bitter overtone. Cultivated Gynostemma contains around 4 percent to 5 percent gypenosides.

Gynostemma is rare in America in bulk form and is mostly available prepackaged. Most of the world's supply is sold to Japan or domestically in China. Mountain-grown wild Gynostemma is considerably more expensive than the farm-grown variety because it is more potent and much more rare. Mountain-grown wild Gynostemma is the connoisseur's choice, whenever possible. This is one of the great health products available in the world today.

Preparation and Utilization: Consuming Gynostemma will not result in any side effects even if taken in considerable quantities over a long period of time. It is an ideal herb to take on a daily basis. Since it is available in the American market as both tea and concentrated powders in capsules, it is easy to consume. It is suitable for both the sick and the healthy, for young and old, for males and females. Children can drink it at will. One cup of Gynostemma tea or two capsules of concentrated powder (about 1,000 mg) a day will have many benefits. I drink two or more cups of Gynostemma tea every day religiously. Twice this amount will not be harmful. Remember that this is at the top of the list of the greatest herbs in the world. I recommend a wonderful tea called Spring Dragon Tea made with Gynostemma and a number of other major tonics, including Lycium and Astragalus.

Some people prefer consuming standardized extracts. Gynostemma saponins, the gypenosides, are available in some products. Recommended doses for gypenosides ranges from 25 to 200 mg per day.

Contraindications: None. Gynostemma and gypenosides are very safe for consumption.

LYCIUM FRUIT

Pharmaceutical Name: Fructus Lycii
Treasures: *Yin jing* and Blood
Atmospheric Energy: Neutral
Taste: Sweet
Organ Associations: Liver, Kidneys, and Lungs
Treasure Rating: ★★★★★

Qualities Attributed to the Fruit: This delicious fruit is very widely used throughout Asia as a superb *yin jing* and blood tonic. It is one of the most popular herbs in the world. Regular consumption of Lycium is believed to lead to a long, vigorous, and happy life. And it is said that prolonged consumption of Lycium will promote cheerfulness and brighten the spirit. Lycium has long been used as a longevity herb. It is believed to fortify the system against disease and to provide the energy to overcome difficult obstacles.

Lycium is said to brighten the eyes and improve vision. It is the primary tonic to vision in Chinese herbalism. Lycium strengthens the legs and has long been a favorite herb of Chinese martial artists and athletes. It has been tested as an antiobesity drug. Patients were given thirty grams each morning and each afternoon to be made into a tea. Most patients lost significant weight.

Lycium is commonly used by first-trimester mothers to prevent morning sickness. Fifty grams of Lycium is boiled along with fifty grams of Scutellaria for thirty minutes. Drinking this tea is a quick and effective remedy for morning sickness.

Lycium is one of the fundamental sexual tonic herbs in Chinese herbalism, especially when blended with *yang* tonic herbs such as Deer Antler, Morinda, and Cordyceps, with *qi* tonics such as Astragalus and Ginseng, and with astringent herbs such as Schizandra and Cornus. Lycii berries are widely believed to increase sexual fluids and enhance fertility.

It is said in China that eating a handful of Lycii berries a day will make you happy for the entire day. Such a practice has a cumulative effect. Eventually, you can't stop smiling.

Fresh Ning Xia Lycium has the highest content of beta-carotene among all foods on earth. Beta-carotene can be transformed into vitamin A under the influence of human liver enzymes. Therefore, vitamin A ultimately plays a major influence in Lycium's actions. Lycium's function on the eyes is related to this factor. In addition, Lycium is rich in zeaxanthin, another carotenoid phytonutrient closely related to beta-carotene which is a superb lipid peroxidase inhibitor.

Lycium's vitamin B_1 and B_2 contents are significant, and the vitamin C content of freeze-dried Lycium has been measured to be 73 mg/100 g. Lycium contains eighteen kinds of amino acids, of which eight are indispensable for the human body. Fifty percent of Lycium's amino acids are free amino acid. Lycium contains numerous trace minerals, of which the main ones are zinc, iron, and copper. Mature fruits contain about 11 mg of iron per 100 g. Lycium is rich in other trace minerals as well. It contains significant amounts of calcium, germanium, selenium, and phosphorus, plus small quantities of many others. Lycium also contains flavonoids, which, due to their antioxidant activity, protect cell membranes.

Lycium contains a range of polysaccharides that have pharmacological effects on lymphocytes and have been shown to improve immunity. Lycium has been shown to have a double-direction, regulatory effect on T lymphocytes and B lymphocytes in test animals. When Lycium extract was provided to twenty elderly people, once a day for three weeks, more than two-thirds of the patients' T cell transformation functions tripled, and the activity of the patients' white cell interleukin-2 doubled. In addition, the results showed that the spirit and optimism of all the patients increased significantly, appetite improved in 95 percent of the patients, 95 percent slept better, and 35 percent at least partially recovered their sexual function.

Varieties and Grading: Because of Lycium's great fame over many, many centuries, it has been collected and cultivated in almost every region of China, where it grows on hillsides and ridges. The best Lycium grows in cool-climate areas. Lycium is collected in the summer and autumn when the fruit is mature.

Though there are several varieties of Lycium, the primary variety is called Ning Xia Lycium. This Lycium is the preferred herb of herbal connoisseurs. It is big, has thick fruit meat, has few seeds, and its taste is sweet and exquisite. Ning Xia Lycium is further graded according to size, larger ones selling for considerably more than smaller ones. The larger ones tend to be sweeter and have a juicier texture. They also have more powerful herbal activity.

At the herb shop, you may select your Lycium by looking at it, feeling it, and tasting it. It should have a uniform red-orange color that is not too bright and not too dark. Some suppliers in Asia dye the fruit red to make it more attractive to naive buyers. It should not have any dark fruit mixed in—dark fruit is oxidized and spoiled. The fruit should be firm and not mushy. Mushy fruit is spoiled. Larger fruit is best. Always taste Lycium before you buy it. It should be delectable. Great Lycium is very sweet and a total pleasure to eat raw or cooked.

Preparation and Utilization: High-quality Lycium is delicious and may be eaten as a snack. Most frequently, it is used in formulas. Combine it with Prepared Rehmannia to strengthen *jing*, nourish Kidney *yin*, and build blood. Combine with Ginseng to strengthen the Heart and Kidneys. Or combine with Schizandra to tonify Kidney and Liver *yin* and strengthen *jing*.

Contraindications: Lycium has absolutely no toxicity. However, it should not be used in the case of a fever due to an infection, or if you are suffering from Spleen deficiency with diarrhea.

MORINDA ROOT

Pharmaceutical Name: Radix Morindae

Treasures: *Jing*

Atmospheric Energy: Sweet

Taste: Pungent and sweet

Organ Associations: Kidneys

Treasure Rating: ★★★★½

Qualities Attributed to the Root: Morinda is an excellent *yang jing* tonic. It is considered to be highly nutritious and is used in superior tonic formulas for strengthening the body. It is widely used in Primal Essence formulations, often as the main ingredient, and sometimes secondarily to *yang* tonics of animal origin, such as Deer Antler, Cordyceps, Sea Dragon, and/or Gecko.

Morinda is often used to increase sexual strength in men and women. It is used for impotence, premature ejaculation, soreness of the lower back and knees, and infertility. In this case, it would be combined with other *yang* herbs and *qi* tonics.

It is used by women for infertility and frigidity. It would be combined with Ginseng or Codonopsis, Astragalus, Dang Gui, White Peony, Lycium, Schizandra, and so forth. It can be used for irregular menstruation, pain and cold sensation in the lower abdomen, and chronic fatigue, especially when combined with these same tonic herbs plus Cinnamon Bark, a warming herb.

Morinda is widely believed in China to increase mental power. It is also considered to be beneficial to the heart. And like many other *yang* tonic herbs, it has been shown to be effective in lowering high blood pressure.

It is a superb athletes' herb and ranks among the most important vitalizing herbs of the tonic system. It is one of the finest *yang jing* tonics, since it is not only powerful but extremely well tolerated by almost everyone. It is considered a major longevity herb and is a regular ingredient in Daoist formulations.

Varieties and Grading: Really good Morinda is large, very pliable, and slightly moist. Poor-quality Morinda is small, brittle, and tasteless.

Preparation and Utilization: Morinda is a premium herb that may be used by itself but is most often found in combination with other tonic herbs. Combine with Ginseng, Cistanches, Lycium, and Cuscuta Seed to tonify Kidney *yang* and to treat impotence, premature ejaculation, infertility, frigidity, irregular menstruation. Or combine with Eucommia Bark, Dipsacus, and Drynaria to treat soreness of the lower back and knees.

Contraindications: Not to be used in cases of *yin* deficiency with excessive fire, or in cases of damp heat.

SCHIZANDRA

Pharmaceutical Name: Fructus Schizandrae
Treasures: *Jing, qi,* and *shen*
Atmospheric Energy: Warm
Taste: Sour and sweet with salty, pungent, and bitter overtones
Organ Associations: Enters all twelve meridians
Treasure Rating: ★★★★★

Qualities Attributed to the Fruit: Chinese women have historically held Schizandra in very high favor, especially the women of the imperial court and other women who practiced the art of beauty, because of its beauty-enhancing qualities. Both men and women used it to promote vigor and alertness.

According to an ancient story, there was a gentleman named Huai Nan Gong who had been taking Schizandra for sixteen years. As a result, he had the complexion of a "Jade Girl" (a way of expressing beauty in Chinese). Legend has it that Huai Nan Gong would stay dry in water and unburned in fire. This story shows that Schizandra was believed capable of maintaining a human body's beauty and strength and protecting the body, particularly the skin, from harm due to the elements.

Schizandra develops the primary energies of life and is thus of great use to anyone who consumes it. Schizandra generates vitality and radiant beauty when used regularly for some time. It is a safe and powerful tonic herb which is mildly calming and possesses pain-alleviating properties. If used for one hundred days successively, Schizandra is said to purify the blood, sharpen the mind, improve memory, rejuvenate the Kidney energy (especially the sexual functions in both men and women), and cause the skin to become radiantly beautiful.

The very name of Schizandra in Chinese tells us a great deal about the qualities of this herb. *Wu wei zi* means "five-taste fruit." Schizandra possesses all five of the classical tastes (sour, bitter, sweet, spicy, and salty) and thus the essence of all five of the elemental energies (Wood, Fire, Earth, Metal, and Water). Schizandra is respected as a health-providing tonic in the same class with Ginseng and Ganoderma.

Schizandra was routinely used by Daoists because of its life-strengthening power, because it empowered the mind, and because of its benefit to the Kidneys and Lungs. Daoists appreciated it because it helped to develop their spiritual power. In addition to all five elemental energies, it contains all Three Treasures in abundance and enters all twelve meridians. Master Sung Jin Park considered it to be the quintessential herbal substance.

Schizandra is said to increase the Water *qi* in the Kidneys. In particular, it is said to vastly increase the "water of the genital organs," referring to the sexual fluids. Schizandra is said to promote the production of semen and is famous for its ability to prevent premature ejaculation, relieve sexual fatigue, and increase the sexual staying power in men. It is thus an ingredient in the vast majority of men's sexual tonics in Asian herbalism.

Women benefit from the same capacity to increase Water *qi* of the Kidneys. Schizandra is said to increase circulation in and sensitivity of the female genitals. Many women claim increased genital warmth and sensation after using Schizandra for a period of time. The Chinese sexual classics claim that continuous use by a woman will increase the amount of "female elixir," a euphemism for vaginal secretions, during intercourse. On the other hand, Schizandra is used clinically to help counteract vaginal discharge.

For both men and women, Schizandra is considered to have aphrodisiac qualities, especially when combined with other Kidney-tonifying herbs like Lycium, Cistanches, Deer Antler, and Epimedium. Furthermore, Schizandra is one of the most important *astringent* herbs used in Chinese herbalism. An astringent herb conserves fluids, and in the case of Schizandra, it tends to contain sexual fluids until the appropriate time of release. Thus, consuming Schizandra for a period of time, one tends to build up sexual fluids.

Schizandra is widely used to beautify the skin and to protect it from the damaging effects of the sun and wind. Due to Schizandra's astringent quality, the skin tends to hold its moisture and becomes full and beautiful. It has always been very popular with the wealthy men and women of China because of its youth-preserving and rejuvenating effects. It is said that those who use Schizandra consistently will remain youthful in both appearance and physiology. I have seen the benefits of this herb with my own eyes hundreds of times. People who start taking Schizandra regularly all change for the better. Their skin virtually glows and becomes clear and fine after several months.

This herb is considered to be one of the premium mind tonics of herbalism. It is used to sharpen concentration, improve memory, and increase alertness. Yet, unlike caffeinelike stimulants, Schizandra does not produce nervousness. In fact, some people consider Schizandra mildly "calming" while producing wakefulness and improved focus.

Schizandra is one of the primary detoxifying herbs used in Chinese herbalism. It helps detoxify the liver. It does not have the side effects that are associated with many of the "medicinal," or "inferior," liver-cleansing herbs. It is believed that by taking Schizandra regularly, it is possible to rid the body of toxins before they have a chance to do serious damage. Schizandra, especially alcohol extracts, is widely believed to protect the liver from damage due to poisons, as well as the by-products of living.

Schizandra is considered to be one of the premier adaptogens. Just like Ginseng, Acanthopanax, and Gynostemma,

Schizandra increases resistance of the body and mind against nonspecific stimuli. It can protect the body from damage due to extreme or chronic stress. In particular, it can protect the adrenals and prevent atrophy due to extreme stress.

Schizandra has been demonstrated in laboratory animals and in humans to have a stimulant action on the central nervous system. The herb works directly on the nervous tissue. Many studies now indicate that Schizandra actually has a powerful balancing, or regulating, action on the central nervous system. It can result in accurate and optimal balancing between the excitatory and inhibitory control functions of the cerebral cortex.

It has been demonstrated that human intellectual activity can be enhanced and work efficiency increased by consuming Schizandra. Various tests have shown that moderate therapeutic doses can improve various activities requiring concentration, fine coordination, sensitivity, and endurance. The tests in humans confirming Schizandra's efficacy in these areas range from threading needles to running marathons.

Human studies have also shown that Schizandra can improve vision, even enlarging the field of vision, and can improve hearing. It also improves the discrimination ability of the skin receptors. It has been determined that this increased sensitivity is due to improved function of the central nervous system's ability to analyze data flowing to it from the peripheral sensors.

Schizandra has been shown to have significant respiratory-strengthening capacity. It can cause the breathing to be both deeper and more powerful. Schizandra also has significant expectorant and antitussive action.

It has also been shown to have significant liver-protecting effects. It can promote the regeneration of liver tissue and promotes protein and nucleic acid syntheses. It is believed that the protective action of Schizandra is partly due to its ability to promote the regeneration of mitochondria in hepatic cells. It can also improve the function of the cell membrane, lowering its permeability, which in turn minimizes enzyme leakage into the bloodstream.

Varieties and Grading: There are two varieties of Schizandra: Northern and Southern. Northern Schizandra is generally considered to be superior to the Southern variety. It is stronger-tasting and more potent. Virtually all Northern Schizandra is collected wild in the mountains and hills away from cities and industrial areas.

The skin and meat of the Schizandra fruit are sweet and sour, the core is pungent and bitter, the whole fruit salty. The fruit, which matures in the fall, is a beautiful, radiant violet-red. The plant grows by entwining itself around low trees in dense areas where forest and grassland meet. In my experience searching for Schizandra in northern China, I have always found that Schizandra grows in relatively inaccessible areas, often near cliffs and streams.

High-quality Schizandra, as we see it in American herb shops, is dried and dark purple with some pinkish tone left. Freshly dried Schizandra has a luster, and the flesh is still plump and tender and has a very pleasant sweet-sour aroma. If the fruit is dark black or brown, or has white patches everywhere, it is probably too old to be fully useful. With experience you will be able to select premium Schizandra with your eyes closed. Fresh Schizandra has a smooth, sweet, highly aromatic fragrance, and the fruit has a wonderful flavor.

Be careful to select good Schizandra. Schizandra may be stored for years before it is sold in herb shops. I have seen Schizandra that is barely recognizable. It was shriveled, black, and lifeless. This Schizandra would be herbally useless. Keep the Schizandra in a tightly closed container in a dark closet, or better yet, refrigerate it. When you find great Schizandra, stock up—it's the quintessence of everything good about tonic herbalism.

Preparation and Utilization: Schizandra contains tannin, which can be difficult on the digestive system, especially if one's stomach and digestive system are weak. Tannin, being water-soluble, can be removed from the Schizandra by soaking it for several hours before using. Most herb shops now presoak Schizandra. Ask your herbalist if this has been done. If not, soak it.

To make a simple tea out of Schizandra, add a handful to three or four cups of water. The exact amount is not important—you can adjust it to your liking. Add a few slices of Licorice Root (after you have made the tea a few times, you will know exactly how much to add to suit your taste). If you like, add a handful of Lycium—this creates a great tonic beverage. Bring the tea to a boil and allow to simmer for fifteen minutes. Do not overcook, as overcooking destroys both the flavor and some of the beneficial constituents in Schizandra. Drink this tea daily for one hundred days to cleanse your Liver, to purify your blood, to sharpen your mind, to beautify your skin, to build Kidney *jing*, and to produce superb sexual energy and "boudoir abundance." Besides being a marvelous tonic, this tea is delicious—quite suitable for serving to friends. Schizandra is a longevity herb and can be safely consumed indefinitely.

Schizandra may be consumed alone, but it is most commonly combined with other tonic herbs. Combine with Prepared Rehmannia and Lycium to tonify the Kidneys and Liver and to promote the production of hormones. Combine with Licorice Root to cleanse the Liver to Lungs. Or blend with Ganoderma to protect the Liver and to strengthen the mind.

Contraindications: None.

POLYGONUM

Pharmaceutical Name: Radix Polygonum multiflorum
Treasures: *Yin jing* and Blood
Atmospheric Energy: Warm
Taste: Bitter, sweet, and pungent
Organ Associations: Liver and Kidneys
Treasure Rating: ★★★★★

Qualities Attributed to the Processed Tuber: Prepared Polygonum is one of the most important and widely used Chinese tonic herbs. It shares the position as the primary Essence tonic of Chinese herbalism with Lycium. It is widely known by its Chinese name, He Shou Wu, and sometimes as Fo Ti (a misnomer).

Polygonum is tonic to the Kidney and Liver functions. It is a potent and surefire *yin* tonic. As such, it strengthens the tendons, ligaments, and bones and prevents premature aging. It reputedly has the capacity to return gray hair to black. This is its most famous attribute and it is widely used throughout Asia for this purpose.

It is also capable of increasing sperm and making the ova more vital. It is therefore considered to be a primary fertility-enhancing herb. Many men have claimed that consuming Polygonum has noticeably increased their sperm production. One client of mine, who was trying to impregnate his wife, told me that after taking Polygonum for one month his sperm count had tripled, according to lab tests. Polygonum is likewise known for increasing fertility in women. Traditionally, this herb has been said to increase *jing* and blood. Both men and women attempting to have children take it.

Another attribute of the herb, associated with its Kidney and Liver tonic effects, is its ability to strengthen the lower back, the knees, and tendons, ligaments, and bones throughout the body. Thus Polygonum is useful not only for maintaining youthfulness but also for providing strength to the body. It is also used to strengthen muscle. Polygonum is therefore very widely used by athletes and martial artists in Asia. It is a perfect *yin jing* tonic for the athletically inclined, providing strength, resilience, and stamina to the body. Alone, or properly combined with other tonic herbs, Polygonum is also an ideal longevity-promoting, antiaging tonic herb.

Research has demonstrated that Polygonum can significantly increase superoxide dismutase (SOD) activity. SOD is a powerful natural antioxidant and free-radical scavenger that has been demonstrated to have powerful antiaging benefits in humans. Polygonum also inhibits beta-monoamine oxidase (ß-MAO). Both of these factors contribute to the antiaging effects of this herb.

Polygonum has been demonstrated to help strengthen the membranes of erythrocytes (red blood cells) and to promote the growth and development of these cells. Traditionally, Polygonum is considered an ideal and potent blood tonic.

Varieties and Grading: There are two varieties of Polygonum sold on the Chinese market: prepared and unprepared. Prepared Polygonum is tonic, with the properties described above. Unprepared Polygonum functions quite differently. It is a laxative, which is also used to treat sores, constipation, and acne. It is not to be confused with the prepared Polygonum.

Polygonum is prepared by boiling it in a soup of black beans. This preparation changes the characteristic of the herb.

The older the tuber, the higher the quality of the herb. Typical Polygonum is not very old these days. Good Polygonum should be at least four years old. Older Polygonum is available to those who seek it, and this older stock is far superior; it not only tastes much better but is much more potent. It is invariably prepared more carefully. Generally, it is sliced thinly and laid out neatly for sale. Befriend your herbalist so that he or she gives you the old Polygonum. It is fairly rare and therefore will cost more, but since Polygonum is inexpensive, even the old stuff is cheap relative to its value as a life-enhancing tonic.

Preparation and Utilization: Polygonum is found in a large variety of products. It is most commonly the primary herb in Essence-building, blood-tonifying longevity formulas. Remember that there are different grades of this herb, and the quality of a product is dependent upon the selection of raw material.

Combine with Ginseng root and Dang Gui to build blood, tonify *yin* and *yang*, and increase *qi*. Or combine with Lycium and Cornus to tonify the Kidneys, strengthen the sexual organs, and calm the nerves. A powerful combination is to blend with Acanthopanax to build energy, blood, and *jing*. To strengthen the Kidneys, nourish *jing* and blood, strengthen and relieve pain in the lower back and knees, turn the hair dark, and prevent spermaturia, combine with Eucommia, Ligustrum fruit, and Cornus fruit.

Contraindications: Gastrointestinal disturbance is the only side effect associated with Polygonum. Soft stool is the result. However, moderate doses of Polygonum rarely have this effect. The disturbance can be corrected by combining with herbs that remove dampness through the urinary pathway, such as Poria or Atractylodes (red or white).

ASPARAGUS ROOT

Pharmaceutical Name: Radix or Tuber Asparagi Lucidus
Treasures: *Yin jing, qi,* and *shen*
Atmospheric Energy: Cold
Taste: Sweet and bitter
Organ Associations: Lungs, Kidneys, and Heart
Treasure Rating: ★★★★★

Qualities Attributed to the Root: Use of wild Asparagus Root is said to lead to a happy, mild manner, excellent vitality, and beautiful skin. It is said to strike a balance in the internal functions of the body.

It has long been one of the most highly prized *shen* tonic herbs consumed by the holy men living in the mountainous regions of China and Korea. Wild Asparagus is said to open up the Heart center, allowing *shen* to flourish, manifesting as feelings of love, goodwill, patience, and peace of mind. Regular consumption of good-quality Asparagus Root seems to lift a person's spirits in a way that is consistent with the Daoist philosophy of attaining happiness. If you take it for some time, you tend to see things from a broader view, indeed almost an unlimited view. Daoists mention that by consuming wild Asparagus Root a person gains the ability to "fly." This flying is really the ability to rise above things that are limited and mundane, even if they seem very important at the moment. From above, we see things in their true light, as having ups and downs. We can readily perceive the intrinsic unity of good and bad, and right and wrong, which are always only relative and ephemeral. The *shen* quality of wild Asparagus Root affects the Heart of a man or woman. This spiritual ability to "fly" is the freedom of spirit one experiences when one has attained harmony with Dao and is guided by universal love. Those who are seeking spiritual attainment should consume good wild Asparagus whenever it is available.

Wild Asparagus Root is also an important Lung tonic. In common Chinese herbalism, this is the quality most often referred to when discussing this herb. Asparagus Root moistens and purifies the lungs, aiding in our breathing, removing toxins from the respiratory tract, and improving all respiratory functions. It increases the Lungs' ability to extract *qi* from the air we breathe. Asparagus Root is especially useful for those who are exposed to smoke or to dry or smoggy air or who otherwise are experiencing dryness of the lungs and upper respiratory passages.

Prolonged consumption will make the skin soft, supple, and smooth. Beautiful skin is the result of pure blood and healthy lungs.

Wild Asparagus Root promotes the production of Kidney *yin*, and prolonged use is beneficial for sexual weakness. Even though its greatest value is in its "love tonic" attributes, wild Asparagus Root is often used in tonics designed to overcome impotence or frigidity on the physical level.

Varieties and Grading: Wild Asparagus is collected in the mountains of northern China and Korea. After collecting it, the roots are cleaned and dried. However, they generally remain moist—in fact, gummy. Good-quality Asparagus Root is soft, chewy, pleasant-tasting, and mildly sweet. Most wild Asparagus Root is yellow, and this is excellent, so long as it is clean, moist, and sweet. But occasionally you can find red wild Asparagus Root. Connoisseurs tend to buy up entire batches of this red Asparagus Root quickly. This is a treasure—it is the herb that the Daoists call the Flying Herb. Buy as much as you can when you see it, because it probably won't be there when you go back to the herb shop again.

Preparation and Utilization: Eat one or two wild Asparagus Roots each day, raw. Eat it slowly—almost let it melt in your mouth. Chew well and breathe deeply. Or cook it with your choice of tonic herbs. It may be combined with a wide range of other tonic herbs. It is common to combine it with Ginseng, Schizandra, and Ganoderma.

Contraindications: Do not use this herb if you do not want to have flying dreams.

CODONOPSIS ROOT

Pharmaceutical Name: Radix Codonopsis
Treasures: *Qi* and Blood
Atmospheric Energy: Neutral
Taste: Sweet
Organ Associations: Spleen and Lungs
Treasure Rating: ★★★★½

Qualities Attributed to the Root: Codonopsis is one of the best-known and most widely used Chinese tonic herbs. It is very mild and has no side effects, yet it is a superb *qi* tonic. It invigorates the Spleen and Lung functions so that *qi* is replenished, and it promotes the production of body fluids. Codonopsis is also an excellent blood tonic and a major immune system tonic.

For many centuries, Codonopsis has been one of China's favorite tonic herbs. It is believed to have an action similar to that of Ginseng, but milder. It is often used in place of Ginseng in formulas that actually call for Ginseng to be used as a main *qi* tonic, especially when the purpose of the formula is to invigorate the Spleen and Lung functions. This is totally acceptable in the Chinese herbal system. However, recent studies have shown that Ginseng and Codonopsis do not share the same chemical basis for their *qi*-building activity. Codonopsis Root has only a small saponin content and does not contain saponins similar to the ginsenosides found in Ginseng. Codonopsis is suited well to women and men who possess excessive *yang* energy already. Codonopsis can always be used as the main *qi* tonic in a person's program when Ginseng is not desired but a *qi* tonic is.

Its blood-building quality makes it especially good for people who are weakened due to illness. Codonopsis is extremely effective at relieving chronic fatigue. Many women use it to build blood, and the Chinese consider Codonopsis to be an herb perfectly suited to nursing mothers, holding that it helps produce milk and that the nutrients in Codonopsis are especially nourishing to babies.

It is rich in immune-stimulating polysaccharides, which are beneficial to everyone. They have been shown to be useful in supporting the immune systems of people with cancer who are using the herbs in conjunction with conventional cancer therapies. Codonopsis can be effective in protecting cancer patients from the side effects of radiation therapy without diminishing its benefits. Codonopsis also has interferon-inducing activity that may be of importance in many immune deficiency conditions, including HIV infection.

Codonopsis is an excellent herb for children. It is mild yet has powerful strengthening effects, especially on the digestive, respiratory, and immune systems. It builds strong muscle in children. Children can start chewing on clean Codonopsis Roots as soon as they have teeth and know how to hold the root to their mouth. It is an excellent teething herb.

Varieties and Grading: Codonopsis is one of the herbs that come in a wide range of grades. Codonopsis grows in the north of China. Both wild and cultivated Codonopsis are available. Wild is superior, and it is more expensive, although it may be somewhat smaller than the cultivated variety. However, superb cultivated Codonopsis is widely available.

Tonic herbalists can easily recognize high-quality Codonopsis. Generally, larger roots are the best. They should be straight and clean, without signs of insect, mold, or fungus contamination. They should be dry on the surface, yet flexible and moist when a piece is chewed. The color should be a light tan. High-quality Codonopsis is sweet-tasting and pleasant. The sweetness in the taste develops after you have chewed on the root for several seconds. Once you've gotten into the tonic herbs a bit, good Codonopsis will taste very pleasant when eaten raw.

Low-grade Codonopsis is much less tasty, and poor Codonopsis has almost no flavor. Because low-grade Codonopsis sells for less, the suppliers spend less time cleaning and preparing it, so it might still be quite dirty. Remember, if you eat an herb like Codonopsis raw, it is best to wash it first to get any remnants of China's good earth off it. Always get the best Codonopsis you can obtain. Poor-quality Codonopsis is of little value to one's health.

Preparation and Utilization: Codonopsis is usually combined with other tonic herbs, but high-quality roots may be eaten, cooked or raw. Use as you would use Ginseng.

Contraindications: None.

DENDROBIUM

Pharmaceutical Name: Herba Dendrobii

Treasures: *Yin jing*

Atmospheric Energy: Slightly cold

Taste: Sweet and lightly salty

Organ Associations: Kidneys, Lungs, and Stomach

Treasure Rating: ★★★★

Qualities Attributed to the Stems and Leaves: Dendrobium is primarily used in China to replenish fluids. It is commonly used in Chinese herbalism as a *yin* tonic which moistens the stomach and Lungs. It can be very effective in treating dryness problems like dry mouth, thirst, stomach pain, mouth sores, sunstroke, and dry lungs and air passages due to dry weather or pollution and smoke. In other words, Dendrobium is used to balance hot, dry conditions, to replace damaged or lost fluids, and to relieve thirst, depression, and deficiency fever as a result of illness.

However, the truly great value of Dendrobium lies elsewhere. Daoist sages, the masters of longevity (and much more), have routinely used Dendrobium as a daily tea for many centuries. Dendrobium is especially useful in quickly and effectively replenishing spent adaptive energy. It has been traditionally used as a daily tea to replace spent *yin jing* of the Kidneys. The Kidneys are considered to be the whole body's reservoir of *yin jing*, so Dendrobium replenishes the whole body. Dendrobium is especially famous for relieving fatigue from overindulgence in sex. Dendrobium increases the sexual fluids in men and women. When combined with Licorice Root, it is made into a tea called honeymooner's tea.

The Daoists say that Dendrobium nourishes the saliva, which they call the Precious Fluid. It can be made into a superb tea for athletes for the purpose of maintaining fluids during exercise or sports.

One last benefit of Dendrobium lies in its beauty-promoting quality. Dendrobium helps keep the skin moist, and constant drinking helps generate beautiful skin.

Varieties and Grading: The best Dendrobium is composed of small threads, usually sold as small wound-up balls. It is quite tart. This wild Dendrobium is expensive but is also extremely powerful. Of the more common commercial grades, large gold or green-gold well-preserved stems and leaves indicate good quality. If the stems and leaves are pulpy, that is excellent. The Dendrobium should not be brittle or crumbly when gently squeezed—this would mean that the Dendrobium is old and will have lost its potency. The white pulp inside the Dendrobium should be fresh-looking and even a bit moist.

Preparation and Utilization: If you are using the wild, string variety, use several grams per pot of tea. If you are using the common commercial grade, which I have found to be excellent through the years, use a good handful per pot of tea. Mix with Licorice Root and other herbs as desired.

Contraindications: None.

EPIMEDIUM

Pharmaceutical Name: Herba Epimedii
Treasures: *Yang jing* and *qi*
Atmospheric Energy: Warm
Taste: Acrid and sweet
Organ Associations: Kidneys and Liver
Treasure Rating: ★★★★

Qualities Attributed to the Leaves: Epimedium is a very powerful *yang* tonic herb. Its power as a *yang* tonic ranks almost with the animal *yang* tonics like Gecko and Deer Antler. This is very unusual for a plant. Its name can be translated, revealingly, as "the herb for the man that likes sex too much, like a goat," or more simply as "passionate goat weed." In general, this is what Epimedium is famous for and the most common purpose for using it. Women, too, often take this herb to increase their sexual drive, but it is usually taken in smaller quantities and combined with women's herbs, which are usually more *yin*. It is used in women's fertility formulas in China.

This herb has been extensively studied in laboratories and clinics in modern China, Korea, and Japan. It has been shown that Epimedium does increase sexual activity in animals and humans. It stimulates the sensory nerves throughout the body, and in particular in the genital region. Epimedium also increases sperm production in men. It has been shown to have a moderate androgen-like influence on the testes, prostate gland, and anal muscles, which will influence sexual desire and activity.

Epimedium lowers high blood pressure but does not reduce it in people with normal blood pressure. It does not influence the blood pressure of people with low blood pressure unless combined with Red Ginseng, in which case blood pressure can be elevated. In China, Epimedium is combined with Morinda to treat hypertension due to menopause.

Perhaps even more important have been the recent discoveries that Epimedium has powerful immune-modulating activity which can support the immune functions of healthy individuals and significantly enhance the immune systems of those who are immune-compromised. Recent confirmed studies have shown that Epimedium has significant anti-HIV activity. Epimedium is officially listed in China as an herb that can help prevent the growth of cancer and has been listed by the Chinese Academy of Medical Sciences as one of an elite group of herbs that slow down aging and promote longevity.

What a remarkable herb! Relaxing, yet sexually invigorating. Not only safe, but an incredible health aid for people concerned about their cardiovascular and immune systems. The only drawback to Epimedium is that it is drying, so it should be used very carefully by those who are too dry or who are otherwise *yin* deficient. First, build up *yin*. If you are only slightly *yin* deficient or wish to protect your *yin*, Epimedium may be taken with *yin* herbs such as Dendrobium and Lycium. People who are in good health may use Epimedium safely and regularly to enhance sexual power and build their immune systems. HIV-infected individuals and other people with weakened immune systems may use Epimedium regularly as long as they are getting a full spectrum of *yin* tonics, *qi* tonics, and blood tonics.

Varieties and Grading: There are a number of varieties of Epimedium. The better grades are prepared with much more care and will cost a little more. Epimedium is an inexpensive herb, so it is better to get the best you can. Little prickly points at the edge of the leaves are considered to be slightly toxic. Better-quality Epimedium will have these edges trimmed off.

Preparation and Utilization: An excellent and simple formula that one can make at home is to combine half a dozen leaves of Epimedium with an ounce each of Schizandra and Lycium. Simmer this in a quart of water until half is boiled away (do not add the Schizandra until the final twenty minutes of cooking). This will strengthen the body by building both the *yin* and *yang* of the Kidneys and Liver. Those who are *yin* deficient may double the Schizandra and Lycium (or reduce the amount of Epimedium by one-half) and may add other *yin*-nourishing herbs such as Polygonum, Dendrobium, Prepared Rehmannia, Dang Gui, Glehnia, Asparagus Root, Ophiopogon, and/or American Ginseng. Such a brew, if most of these herbs were used, would be superb for those who are experiencing deep exhaustion. Those who want more *yang* action may add herbs like Ginseng, Eucommia, Cistanches, Cordyceps, Cnidium, and/or Sea Horse.

You will find Epimedium in commercial formulas designed to enhance libido and the immune system.

Contraindications: Not to be used by men with hyperactive sexual drive. Not to be used over a long period of time by people who are *yin*-deficient and suffer from dryness and heat syndromes.

EUCOMMIA BARK

Pharmaceutical Name: Cortex Eucommia
Treasures: Primarily *yang jing*, but also *yin jing* to a lesser degree
Atmospheric Energy: Warm
Taste: Sweet
Organ Associations: Kidneys and Liver
Treasure Rating: ★★★★★

Qualities Attributed to the Bark: Eucommia is the primary plant source in Chinese herbalism used to tonify the *yang jing* functions of the Kidneys, in particular as it affects the lower part of the body and the skeletal structure. Eucommia is a superb *yang jing* tonic and also nourishes *yin jing*. Because it provides both *yin* and *yang*, it is good for men and women alike and can be used by almost anybody to promote endocrine system and sexual functions, to enhance normal growth, to promote healing, and to strengthen the physical structure and resistance.

Eucommia's first fame is in its Kidney-tonifying effects. It is the primary herb in Chinese tonic herbalism for building a strong, sturdy, flexible skeletal structure. It is used to strengthen the bones, ligaments, and tendons and can be used to help mend damage to these tissues, whether the damage is due to stress, age, or trauma. Eucommia is also the primary herb of choice for lower back and knee problems, including pain, stiffness, dislocation, swelling, and weakness. Eucommia is one of the few herbs in Chinese tonic herbalism that are sufficiently powerful, balanced, and broad-spectrum to be used alone. However, it is generally combined with other tonic herbs in formulations designed to build the *yin* and *yang* of the Kidneys.

As a Kidney tonic, Eucommia is considered an important herb for improving potency in men and fertility in women. It will be found in almost every formula designed for such purposes. Furthermore, Eucommia helps slow down ejaculation.

Eucommia has been used for over a thousand years to ease tension and relieve the symptoms of high blood pressure and is widely used clinically for hypertension. The ability of Eucommia to safely reduce high blood pressure has been well established by many animal and human clinical studies. Eucommia was found to contain hypotensive compounds in 1974 at the University of Wisconsin; hypotensive compounds exist in both the bark and leaves. It may be used along with conventional Western drugs if desired, as it is in Asia, since Eucommia is very mild and has no known negative interactions with drugs or adverse side effects.

The hypotensive action of the herb has been investigated in several large clinical studies. Although the blood-pressure-reducing effects of Eucommia are not as powerful or quick as the effects of reserpine, Eucommia is more effective in reducing the symptoms of high blood pressure. Eucommia has also been shown to have a mild diuretic action.

Eucommia markedly reduced cholesterol absorption in laboratory animals. It also had mild sedative and anti-inflammatory action in pharmacological experiments. Experimental results indicated that one of the anti-inflammatory mechanisms of Eucommia involves enhancement of the adrenocortical function. This supports the traditional theory that Eucommia tonifies the Kidney functions, which are now known to involve adrenocortical function.

Decoctions of this herb have been shown to have powerful effects on the immune systems of various laboratory animals. In particular, it appears that Eucommia significantly enhances phagocytic action. Phagocytosis involves the clearing away of foreign material from the bloodstream by the white blood cells. In this particular action, Eucommia proved to be as powerful as Astragalus and Codonopsis, which have been proved to have powerful immunological activity in animals and humans. Many studies have shown that Eucommia potentiates the immunologic functions of the body.

Varieties and Grading: Eucommia Bark is peeled from trees that are ten years old or older. A small patch of the bark is peeled off the tree each year so as not to harm the tree, which can grow to be over a hundred years old. The older the bark, the thicker it becomes.

Inside the bark is a pure white latex. Eucommia is the only temperate zone rubber tree. This latex is noticeably elastic. If you gently break a piece of Eucommia Bark and stretch it slightly, the latex will stretch. This rubber is believed to confer strength to connective tissue and is considered to be part of Eucommia's active ingredients. The thicker and stronger this latex, the better the quality of the specimen. Therefore, in purchasing Eucommia, select (1) thick pieces, since these are older, and (2) Eucommia with the most white latex.

Preparation and Utilization: Eucommia usually comes presliced. You will note small transverse slices across the bark at quarter-inch intervals. These slices expose the inside of the bark, including the latex. This is standard practice. If the Eucommia you purchase does not come sliced, have the herb shop slice it for you, or you will have to slice it yourself. The inside must be exposed to the cooking water in order to be properly and efficiently cooked.

Eucommia may be used as an ingredient in any *yang* tonic formulation. It is often combined with Ginseng and other *qi* tonics as well. Combine with Ginseng, Epimedium, Sea Dragon, and Gecko to tonify Kidney *yang* and to build sexual energy. Combine with Lycium, Morinda, Achyranthes, and Cnidium Seed to strengthen the lower back and knees.

Contraindications: There has never been a case of overdosing on Eucommia recorded in the literature (over a period of more than 2,500 years).

LICORICE ROOT

Pharmaceutical Name: Radix Glycyrrhizae

Treasures: *Qi*

Atmospheric Energy: Neutral

Taste: Sweet

Organ Associations: Spleen, Stomach, and Lungs

Treasure Rating: ★★★★

Qualities Attributed to the Root: Licorice Root is used in more formulations than any other herb in Chinese herbalism. It is considered to be the quintessential "servant" herb. Its sweet and pleasant flavor helps make some unsavory formulations palatable, and otherwise bland-tasting formulations pleasant.

It is believed that Licorice Root "harmonizes" the ingredients in an herbal formulation, eliminating harshness of action and promoting smooth activity of the herbs. It is therefore called the Great Harmonizer and is extremely important in the Chinese herbal system, both tonic and medicinal. The herb is powerful, and small doses are usually sufficient to achieve excellent results.

Licorice is an excellent *qi* tonic. It increases vital energy. This herb is frequently used to strengthen the digestive and metabolic functions. It aids in the assimilation of nutrients and thus contributes to the building of blood. Licorice helps build strong muscle tissue. It is thus widely used by athletes, dancers, and other physically active people. It is used as an ingredient in numerous *qi* tonic formulations as both a *qi* tonic and the harmonizing ingredient.

Licorice Root is often used as an anti-inflammatory agent, with an action similar to hydrocortisone. Glycyrrhizin and glycyrrhetinic acid, the two primary active ingredients of Licorice Root, are believed to be the components responsible for this activity. It is useful for all sorts of inflammation, but usually it depends on the other herbs in a formula to determine where the formula will act.

This herb has a reputation as an excellent expectorant in the case of lung congestion. Furthermore, it is widely used as a tea to help relieve sore throat and pharyngolaryngitis. Millions of smokers use it to soothe their dry throats, since Licorice Root improves secretion of the throat mucosa. It is also used as an ingredient in teas by singers, public speakers, and others who utilize their vocal cords excessively.

Licorice Root has acquired the name in China of the Great Detoxifier. It is considered to be one of the primary detoxifying herbs in the Chinese herbal arsenal. Low-level consumption of Licorice Root will rid the body of poisons that would otherwise accumulate and cause disease or functional disorder if not cleaned out. In particular, it cleans the blood and the Liver. Though there are many detoxifying agents used in Chinese herbalism, most of them are harsh. Licorice Root, on the other hand, is mild and, for most people, devoid of negative side effects. It can be used preventively, which makes it more generally useful then medicinal herbs.

Licorice Root is also used as an antispasmotic. When combined with White Peony Root, it is a superb antispasmotic. These two herbs work synergistically to relax both smooth muscle and striated muscle. It is especially known for relieving cramps in the calves and feet.

Another use for which Licorice Root is famed is the relief of gastric and duodenal ulcers. Numerous reports confirm Licorice Root's traditional use as an antiulcer agent. It has shown significant inhibition on experimental ulcers as well as in human clinical settings. It protects the mucosa against damage. One mechanism is by inhibiting abnormal gastric secretion by the gastric mucosal cells. FM 100 is the primary component involved in this action. It is especially effective when combined with herbs like Gynostemma and White Peony, which themselves help relieve ulcers.

Licorice Root is an indispensable component of the Chinese herbal system. It has powerful tonic benefits and at the same time has a wide range of healing effects. The trick in using Licorice Root lies in watchful moderation. Don't use too much—it's unnecessary, and excessive quantities can cause water retention. Small doses are very unlikely to have any results but excellent ones.

Varieties and Grading: Large, very sweet Licorice Root is the best. Very high-quality Licorice Root, when sliced, has a smoother, finer texture than cheap, low-grade Licorice. Good Licorice Root is pleasant to chew. Licorice Root is a soft wood that becomes pulpy when chewed. Cheaper Licorice Root tends to be more splintery when chewed and doesn't taste as good. Sometimes small, splintery Licorice Root is quite sweet. This type of Licorice is fine for extraction, but the larger Licorice Root has better chemical harmony and is simply better in most cases. All Licorice Root is inexpensive, and it goes a long way because you will be using small quantities, so purchase the best you can find.

Preparation and Utilization: Licorice Root is an adjunctive herb. Small amounts may be added to almost any herbal brew you prepare to sweeten the flavor and enhance the activity of the other herbs.

Contraindications: Large doses of Licorice Root can result in side effects associated with the adrenocorticomimetic action of the herb. The symptoms associated with Licorice Root include edema and hypertension. Patients prone to, or suffering from, these disorders should use Licorice Root only sparingly, as a low-level adjunctive herb in herbal formulations, or they should use deglycyrrhinated Licorice Root extracts. In addition, they should seek the advice of their health practitioner. Elderly patients in particular should use Licorice Root sparingly and under the supervision of an herbalist.

NOTOGINSENG ROOT

Pharmaceutical Name: Radix Notoginseng or Radix Pseudoginseng
Treasures: Blood
Atmospheric Energy: Slightly warm
Taste: Bitter and slightly sweet
Organ Associations: Heart
Treasure Rating: ★★★★

Qualities Attributed to the Root: The Notoginseng plant looks similar to Siberian Ginseng and contains saponins similar to those of Panax Ginseng. It is commonly called by its Chinese name, San Qi. Li Shi Chen, China's most renowned herbalist, said that "San Qi is more valuable than gold," and since that time this herb has often been referred to as "Not to Be Exchanged for Gold." It has also been called the Miracle Root for the Preservation of Life.

Prepared (Steamed) San Qi: Steamed Notoginseng is a very efficacious blood tonic. It is used to strengthen the body and to promote growth, recovery, and healing. It also reduces blood LDL (low-density, "bad" cholesterol) levels and is widely used in China as a longevity herb based on its cardiotonic action. Because of the root's strong bitter flavor, it is not used as often as a blood tonic in teas and soups as it would be if it tasted better. However, in this modern age of capsules, steamed Notoginseng has become one of the great blood tonics known to humankind.

Pharmacological studies have demonstrated that Notoginseng has many physiological functions. It has bipolar, double-direction effects on several fundamental physiological functions, including the nervous system, various aspects of the endocrine system, the immune system, and the cardiovascular system. It has shown anti-inflammatory and antihepatitis effects. It protects the liver and has anticarcinogenic activity on many strains of cancer. It has shown antiaging activity in laboratory animals.

Notoginseng Root is rich in saponins. It contains more than twelve saponins, and approximately 12 percent of the root extract is saponins. The primary saponins are very similar, or in some cases identical, to ginsenosides derived from Panax Ginseng. It also contains many kinds of amino acids and trace elements. In fact, Notoginseng is richer in active constituents than either Panax or American Ginseng. Steamed San Qi is rich in iron, calcium, and flavonoids. It appears that these substances provide raw material for the synthesis, in humans, of major adrenal hormones such as cortisol and reproductive hormones such as testosterone, estrogen, and progesterone. It has been found to promote nonspecific RNA to deploy amino acids to form gamma globulin, which acts as an antibody for the control and prevention of a broad spectrum of diseases.

The actions of this herb on the cardiovascular system have been extensively investigated. Panax Notoginseng has been shown to dilate the coronary artery and to increase coronary blood flow and thus provides more blood to the cardiac muscle in humans. The herb reduces cardiac load and lowers arterial pressure. It improves collateral microcirculation in and around damaged heart tissue in humans.

Raw San Qi: Some of the most significant and astounding research findings revolve around *raw* Notoginseng's ability to positively affect the heart and its tributaries. Extensive Chinese research indicates that raw (unsteamed) Notoginseng increases blood flow in the coronary artery (the artery that supplies the heart itself with blood) and increases the consumption of oxygen in the middle muscular layer of the heart. This results in the lowering of blood pressure and in improving regularity of the heartbeat. This has led to the conclusion by Chinese medical researchers and doctors that Notoginseng can prevent insufficiency caused by stagnation of blood in the heart.

Notoginseng has been found to clinically relieve chest pain and the feeling of oppression in the chest due to angina pectoris, resulting from coronary insufficiency. Raw Notoginseng is widely used clinically in Asian countries for angina pectoris and other coronary disease. It is often given in conjunction with Western-style drugs under a doctor's supervision. It is also used to reduce triglycerides and the cholesterol levels in the blood and coating the arteries.

The herb, both raw and steamed, has been shown to have hemostatic, anticoagulant, and platelet-function-suppressing action in animals and in humans. The uncooked raw herb in particular has an extremely potent hemostatic effect—that is, it stops all sorts of bleeding, both internal and external, quickly and effectively. The finely ground powder of raw Notoginseng can be used alone and applied externally to wounds to stop bleeding. It is extremely effective. It is often mixed in liniments to be applied to bruises to disperse the clotting and relieve swelling and pain.

Varieties and Grading: If you want raw San Qi, you can obtain both capsules and powdered San Qi at Chinese herb shops. Sliced raw San Qi can also be obtained from the herb shop and ground in a coffee grinder. Whole San Qi is generally available at Chinese herb shops as well. My view is that these are usually the best San Qi available. Larger roots are considered premium. They are hard, so you should have the herb shop crush them or slice them for you for efficient cooking or easy grinding.

Preparation and Utilization: As a blood tonic or to build strength after surgery or while recovering from an illness, whole roots may be cooked with chicken or with other tonic herbs. (Traditionally, in China, San Qi is almost always cooked with chicken because the chicken eliminates the bitter flavor of the San Qi. The resultant soup is mild and delicious, especially if other vegetables have been added.) Among the tonic herbs, San Qi is one of the least pleasant-tasting. It has a bitter flavor that is difficult to get used to. For this reason, capsules and pills are the best way to take San Qi unless it is a minor ingredient in an herbal formula that overwhelms its flavor.

For those who wish to use raw San Qi to benefit the cardio-vascular system, capsules are best. San Qi is an ingredient in many commercial cardiovascular tonic formulations. As always, if you suffer from heart disease, consult a physician or other primary care practitioner before using raw San Qi.

Contraindications: Notoginseng should never be taken during pregnancy. Notoginseng has the capacity to "dissolve" and cause the expulsion of blood clots lodged anywhere in the body. It is especially useful for dissolving and eliminating blood clots in the pelvic basin. However, it has been found that Notoginseng treats an embryo as a blood clot and can therefore result in miscarriage. Raw Notoginseng is much stronger in this regard than steamed Notoginseng.

PEARL

Pharmaceutical Name: Margarita
Treasures: *Shen*
Atmospheric Energy: Cold
Taste: Salty and sweet
Organ Associations: Heart and Liver
Treasure Rating: ★★★★½

Qualities Attributed to Pearl: To many people's surprise, Pearl is not just a mineral. It contains dozens of amino acids (eight of the amino acids cannot be produced in the body but are required for health) and dozens of minerals, including calcium, magnesium, zinc, iron, strontium, copper, selenium, silicon, and titanium.

Various components in Pearl participate in DNA and RNA metabolic activities and can thus promote and accelerate cell renewal. Mucopolysaccharides in Pearl have been shown to prevent wrinkling and to increase libido and sexual potency in humans.

Pearls have a tremendous reputation in China as both a beauty tonic and a *shen* tonic when consumed orally. Recent Chinese medical texts credit Pearl with the ability to relieve uneasiness of the Heart and mind, to benefit reproduction, to relieve "wandering arthritis," to relieve internal fever, to clear sputum, to remove visual obstacles and improve eyesight, to promote muscle development, and to invigorate blood circulation.

As a beauty tonic, Pearl is hard to beat as a nutritional supplement. The components in Pearl powder help heal blemishes and maintain the health of the skin by participating in the metabolic activities of the skin. Pearl promotes the regeneration of new cells and makes the skin smooth, fine, elastic, and naturally beautiful. High-quality Pearl powder can promote the activities of the important natural antioxidant enzyme SOD and can help prevent the development of melanin, which causes freckles and dark patches on the skin. It can help prevent the skin from becoming old-looking, wrinkled, and sagging. This is partly due to its stimulation of SOD activity and partly to other capacities and phytonutrients. Consistent use of Pearl powder can eliminate blemishes such as colored spots and even pimples and boils. Constant use can help assure that the skin will age much more slowly and that it will not be easily harmed by either time or the elements. Pearl is one of the great secrets of the most beautiful women of the Orient.

Pearl is also a powerful *shen* stabilizer. It is among the elite substances of this type known. It can relieve uneasiness, nervousness, anxiety, and tension. Pearl promotes sound sleep, prevents nerve disorders and nerve weakness, and is commonly used to prevent or overcome fatigue. Consistent use helps a person maintain energy and vitality. It is an ideal *shen* tonic and is the main ingredient in the finest *shen* tonic formulations.

Hydrolyzed Pearl powder, which is Pearl that has been broken down for easy and complete absorption, has been shown in China to help the growth of children's teeth and bones and to improve children's intelligence. Hydrolyzed Pearl has also been shown to be beneficial for habitual constipation, acting quickly, gently, and effectively. Studies indicate that hydrolyzed Pearl can lower blood pressure, increase endurance, and prevent osteoporosis and various cardiovascular diseases. Recent studies indicate that hydrolyzed Pearl is effective in healing inflammation of the uterus.

Varieties and Grading: Basically, there are two types of pearls: natural and cultivated. Natural pearls are much more expensive and are considered to be superior to cultivated pearls for both external, cosmetic use and internal, nutritional use. The natural pearls used in herbalism are very small. The smaller the pearl, the more potent and effective it is as an herb. Some pearls are not much larger than a grain of salt. These very small pearls, which are softer, can be easily crushed and ground into very fine powder, which can be absorbed with relatively high efficiency by the digestive tract. Larger pearls tend to be much harder to grind into fine powder and are thus harder to digest. Small natural pearls are quite expensive, costing between $100 and $1,000 an ounce at Chinese herb shops in Hong Kong or in America.

Cultivated pearls are not considered to be of the same herbal quality as natural pearls. They tend to be large and difficult to grind into fine powder. However, over the last decade a new technology has been developed in China whereby the cultivated pearls are "hydrolyzed." Through modern advanced biochemical technology, Pearl can now be made virtually totally water-soluble. The result is pure *instant* Pearl powder. The solubility rate of this hydrolyzed Pearl is 98 percent, and of this, studies have shown that 95 percent is absorbed into the bloodstream through the digestive tract. This absorbability is approximately four times the bioavailability of normal ground Pearl and double that of the finest-ground natural Pearl. This increased bioavailability and the enormous reduction in cost makes the hydrolyzed Pearl an extraordinary value for all but the richest of herbal consumers—and even for the rich and famous, a blend of hydrolyzed and premium natural Pearl is probably best.

In buying supplements with Pearl powder, be sure that you are buying a brand that you can trust.

If you are buying your own pearls to grind, do not use cultivated pearls unless they are hydrolyzed (dissolvable). Do not buy dissolvable, hydrolyzed Pearl powder from a dealer that you do not know and trust. Some Pearl powders on the market are not real Pearl, or contain Pearl mixed with adulterants. Some of these counterfeits come in lovely packages, but they are worthless. Good Pearl powder costs a little more than the cheaper brands but is well worth the added expense. My advice in buying pearls: Buy high-quality natural Pearl or buy the most expensive hydrolyzed Pearl you can find.

Preparation and Utilization: Pearl can be fed to the skin both through external application and by taking it as a supplement. Many women are familiar with Pearl creams, but few are aware that Pearl is even better utilized by consuming it and letting it nourish the skin through the bloodstream. The best Pearl creams now use hydrolyzed, dissolvable pearl, since it is easily absorbed into the skin. Use according to instructions.

If you buy high-grade natural pearls and have them ground into a fine powder, consuming between two and five grams a month is sufficient to improve the beauty of the skin and to adjust *shen*. Simply place a little of the powder on your tongue and swallow with a drink. If you buy hydrolyzed Pearl powder, consuming between 500 mg (½ g) and one gram per day is usually sufficient to achieve the best results. Be consistent and the results will amaze you.

Contraindications: None. Pearl is extremely safe. Safety studies on hydrolyzed Pearl have shown it to be absolutely harmless. It can be taken by anybody for the course of a lifetime without negative side effects.

PREPARED REHMANNIA

Pharmaceutical Name: Radix Rehmanniae Praparatae
Treasures: *Yin jing* and Blood
Atmospheric Energy: Slightly warm
Taste: Sweet
Organ Associations: Kidneys, Liver, and Heart
Treasure Rating: ★★★★★

Qualities Attributed to the Prepared Root: Rehmannia is said to be the "Kidneys' own food." It is a fundamental Kidney tonic in Chinese tonic herbalism and is considered to be a primary longevity herb. Since antiquity, it has been used in a great many antiaging formulations. It is considered rejuvenating and life-lengthening.

Prepared Rehmannia is a fundamental *yin jing* tonic, providing *yin jing* directly to the Kidneys. It is quick and effective. It is said to benefit sexual functions in men and women and is included in almost every formula that is designed to strengthen reproductive functions, including fertility.

Prepared Rehmannia is a major blood tonic. This is of special importance to women, who always need to rebuild blood. Prepared Rehmannia is said to be warm in nature and thus warms up the uterus in women. A "cold uterus" will result in painful menstruation and infertility.

It is routinely combined with Dang Gui to produce blood. When combined with Dang Gui, Ligusticum, and White Peony, it forms the quintessential women's herbal formula. Prepared Rehmannia is usually combined with *qi* tonics to improve its assimilation. It is also combined with Astragalus, and Deer Antler as well as more common tonic herbs in tonic formulations.

Varieties and Grading: There are two fundamental varieties of Rehmannia used in Chinese herbalism: prepared and raw. Raw

Rehmannia has simply been dried. It has a cold nature and is not particularly tonic (its tonic nature has not been activated). Raw Rehmannia is used primarily in medicinal herbalism to cool down inflammatory conditions. Prepared Rehmannia is highly tonic. It is prepared by soaking in a special blend of wine (which itself has been specially prepared with Amomi and Tangerine Peel) and then steaming and sun-drying. The Rehmannia becomes deep black, soft, and sticky. It is sold in slices in most markets for easy handling. Most Prepared Rehmannia sold in America is of high quality. It will be soft, easily chewed, fine in texture, and very sweet.

Preparation and Utilization: Prepared Rehmannia is never used alone. Combine with Dang Gui and White Peony to build blood and Kidney *yin*. Or combine with Asparagus Root to tonify *yin*, build blood, and calm the Heart. Or combine with Ophiopogon and Cuscuta Seed to tonify the Heart, Kidneys, *jing*, and blood.

Contraindications: Rehmannia is considered to be "greasy" and "slippery," which means that it can cause loose stool in people with weak digestive systems. That is why it should be combined with *qi* tonics. Use cautiously if prone to diarrhea and replace it with Polygonum if loose stools continue to occur.

DANG GUI

Pharmaceutical Name: Radix Angelica Sinensis
Treasures: Blood
Atmospheric Energy: Warm
Taste: Pungent and sweet
Organ Associations: Spleen, Kidneys, and Liver
Treasure Rating: ★★★★½

Qualities Attributed to the Root: Dang Gui is one of the best-known and most widely used herbs in the world. Though it is often described as a women's herb, it is also commonly used by men as a component of a tonic formulation. Dang Gui is most well known for its two primary functions: as a potent and effective blood tonic and as a gynecological regulator.

As a blood tonic, Dang Gui is almost incomparable. Few herbs in the world are either as safe or as potent as a blood tonic. It is used by millions of people to treat common anemia. It can be used after an illness, injury, or surgery to rebuild red blood cells and to increase blood volume. Dang Gui is found in numerous general tonic formulations as part of the blood-building component of the formula. Men as well as women benefit from strong blood.

Dang Gui is Chinese herbalism's most important gynecological herb. It is commonly used by women to build blood. It is most frequently used after a woman's menstrual period has concluded, in order to replenish lost blood. It is used in almost all formulas designed to treat painful menstruation and other menstrual disturbances. It has an analgesic action in the case of dysmenorrhea (painful menstruation), which is attributed to its double-direction, regulating effect on the uterus. Dang Gui is mildly sedative and soothing to nervous disorders and excessive emotionalism.

Dang Gui is routinely used to treat amenorrhea (no menstruation), infertility, premenstrual syndrome, and menopausal distress. It is generally combined with other herbs to suit the condition and the constitution of the woman. These Dang Gui–based formulations are extraordinarily effective and they are safe. Some of these formulations may be consumed as health-promoting tonics. They help regulate the menstrual functions and prevent degeneration of the reproductive system. Therefore, Dang Gui is used in many Chinese youth-preserving formulations.

It is included in most beauty tonics as well. The herb has been found to benefit the complexion by improving circulation in the skin and by detoxifying, thus helping to clear blemishes. It is almost always included in formulations designed to detoxify the skin and is used to treat urticaria, eczema, neurodermatitis, pruritus, vitiligo, rosacea, alopecia, and pigment diseases.

Pharmacological studies indicate that Dang Gui does not have estrogenic action, contrary to earlier reports.

The blood tonic effect of Dang Gui is now attributed to its vitamin B_{12}, folic acid, folinic acid, nicotinic acid, and biotin contents. It is also rich in the metal cobalt, the major element responsible for the hemotinic (blood-enriching) action of B_{12}. Experiments have shown that once vitamin B_{12} loses 0.01 gram of cobalt, its hemotinic effect immediately disappears.

Dang Gui has been found to protect laboratory animals against the symptoms of vitamin E deficiency.

Varieties and Grading: Dang Gui comes in a wide range of qualities. The best Dang Gui is large, clean, and sweet. It has a pleasant yet potent fragrance that smells fresh. Such high-grade Dang Gui comes from north-central China, from provinces such as Gansu and Shanxi. The best Dang Gui has a higher content of volatile oils, accounting for its aroma and flavor. Lower-grade Dang Gui is smaller and not as good-smelling. Poor-quality Dang Gui is not pleasant-smelling or -tasting, or it has little or no aroma. Old Dang Gui that lacks much fragrance or taste is fairly useless.

Preparation and Utilization: Dang Gui may be used alone but is most commonly combined with other herbs. Combine with Ginseng or Codonopsis Root to tonify *yin* and *yang, qi,* and blood. You may also combine with Ligusticum, Prepared Rehmannia, and White Peony to tonify blood and *yin jing,* improve blood circulation, regulate menstrual functions, and relieve menstrual pain. Dang Gui may be combined with Deer Antler to tonify *jing,* blood, and fluids, to fortify the Kidneys, and to sharpen the mind.

Contraindications: Dang Gui should not be used against your doctor's orders. It should not be used by women with breast cancer.

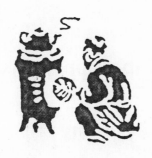

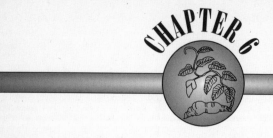

CHAPTER 6

The Supporting Cast of Chinese Herbs

There are a number of very important herbs that are used routinely in the superior herb formulations of China that play primarily a supportive or secondary role in the system. Most of these herbs are supportive tonics, while a few are categorized as general herbs.

THE MAJOR SUPPORTIVE HERBS

BUPLEURUM ROOT

Pharmaceutical Name: Radix Bupleuri
Treasures: None
Atmospheric Energy: Cold
Taste: Bitter
Organ Associations: Liver and Gallbladder
Treasure Rating: None

Qualities Attributed to the Root: Bupleurum Root is one of the most important herbs used in Chinese herbalism. It is not a tonic herb, but it is useful in the tonic system because of its ability to relieve Liver tension and digestive disturbances, and because it is detoxifying and antimicrobial. When combined with other herbs, Bupleurum has the ability to clear stagnation virtually anywhere in the body. It can be used to relieve spasms, muscle tension, lumps, bleeding due to heat, and menstrual irregularity. The essential oil in Bupleurum is responsible for its ability to relieve surface heat.

Bupleurum-based formulations regulate body energy, allowing *qi* to flow freely and steadily. These formulations are often used for relieving blockages in the body and then discharging the toxin safely out of the system. Bupleurum formulas are extremely useful at the early stages of tonic use in helping to establish radiant health, because they assure that the newly abundant energy will flow freely through the body. As time goes by, these formulas become less and less necessary until eventually they only need to be used occasionally, if at all.

Bupleurum is a powerful, cold, detoxifying herb. Since it is not a tonic herb, it has the potential to have side effects if not used carefully. The primary side effect is excessive detoxification in too short a period of time. For this reason, Bupleurum must always be combined with either White Peony or Scutellaria, both of which detoxify the blood and eliminate heat (and any side effects of Bupleurum). They tend to prevent overzealous detoxifying. The toxins will be released more or less unnoticed by the bowels and through perspiration and urination.

Contraindications: Use under the care of an herbalist. May cause rapid detoxification, with symptoms such as headache and anger. In cases of severe toxicity and improperly balanced Bupleurum administration, skin sores can arise.

DIOSCOREA ROOT

Pharmaceutical Name: Rhizoma Dioscoreae
Treasures: *Yin jing* and *qi*
Atmospheric Energy: Neutral
Taste: Sweet
Organ Associations: Kidneys and Spleen
Treasure Rating: ★★★★

Qualities Attributed to the Root: Dioscorea, whose literal name in Chinese is Mountain Medicine, is one of the more widely used tonic herbs. Because the herb has a neutral "atmospheric energy," and therefore is neither hot nor cold, it benefits both the *yin* and the *yang* of the Lungs, Kidneys, and Spleen.

It builds Spleen *qi*, which results in strong digestion and metabolism. It is often combined with Ginseng, White Atractylodes, and Poria to fortify the *qi*-producing power of the digestive tract. Dioscorea is a great herb for people who suffer from loose stool and is very effective at treating many types of diarrhea.

Used with Codonopsis, American Ginseng, Ophiopogon, Schizandra, and other herbs that benefit the Lungs, Dioscorea helps strengthen Lung functioning, which in turn strengthens the whole body.

Dioscorea is a valuable herb in the process of rebuilding and maintaining healthy Kidney functions. It has both *yin jing*–building power and an astringent action that helps consolidate the Kidney energy, preventing "leaking" of fluids. It is widely recommended for the leakage problems that occur as a result of a deficiency of the Kidneys, such as spermatorrhea, leukorrhagia, and frequent urination. It is also often used by people suffering night sweats as a result of general weakness or chronic consumptive illness.

When taken as a tea or with sufficient water, Dioscorea is a superb herb for helping replenish body fluids. It is a powerful herb for treating dehydration due to illness, excessive sweating from physical activity, dry weather, or whatever. Diabetes is a disorder for which Dioscorea is very highly recommended in Asia. The vast majority of Chinese people with diabetes drink a tea of Dioscorea, or a blend of Dioscorea with other herbs, throughout the day to help with the thirst.

Dioscorea is a safe and mild herb that can be used as a nutrient tonic on a regular basis. Being a type of yam, it is often included in food products and used in routine Chinese cooking as a health food. The slices of Dioscorea are quite edible. Dioscorea can easily be crushed or ground into a powder, which makes an excellent ingredient in almost any cooking where flour, grain, or starch might otherwise be used.

Contraindications: Dioscorea should be used only sparingly in cases of abdominal distension due to food stagnancy.

GINKGO BILOBA

Pharmaceutical Name: Folium Ginkgo
Treasures: *Qi*
Atmospheric Energy: Cool
Taste: Bitter
Organ Associations: Heart
Treasure Rating: ★★★

Qualities Attributed to the Standardized Extract of the Leaf: *Ginkgo biloba* is believed to be the oldest living species of tree, dating back nearly 200 million years. The tree itself is capable of a very long life, and individual trees have been reported to have lived over one thousand years.

Ginkgo seed (sometimes called Ginkgo nut) has long been used in Chinese herbalism to clear the lungs of phlegm. It is sometimes used in Chinese cooking. The leaf, however, was not a standard herb in Chinese herbalism until the past decade. But with the advent and popularization of antioxidant theory in recent years, Ginkgo leaf extract has rapidly become one of the most widely used health supplements in the world.

It first gained wide acceptance in Japan and Germany, and has since become very popular in America, Australia, and many other countries. Ginkgo is now one of the most thoroughly studied herbs in the world.

Ginkgo biloba contains flavone-glycosides, including quercetin and proanthocyanidins, which are extremely potent and beneficial antioxidants. In fact, it is the standardized, high-potency extract of Ginkgo (standardized to 24 percent flavone-glycosides) that is most commonly sold in the marketplace. These ginkgo-flavone-glycosides have powerful antioxidant and free-radical scavenging capability. They are considered to be antiaging agents.

Another component of *Ginkgo biloba* is the terpene fraction.

This component has a powerful anti-inflammatory effect. It reduces the stickiness of the blood by inhibiting the platelet-activating factor, which causes platelets to stick together, reducing the flow of blood.

Ginkgo biloba has gained widespread acceptance as a mind tonic. Since it has been determined that Ginkgo increases blood circulation in the brain, it has been accepted as a treatment for memory loss and poor concentration. It is even being used for more serious problems such as cerebrovascular insufficiency, senility, dementia, Alzheimer's disease, vertigo, tinnitus, and dizziness.

It is also being used for peripheral vascular problems, including numbness, impotence, and Raynaud's syndrome, and is being used clinically for hemorrhoids, inflammation, migraines, allergies, and asthma.

Contraindications: None known. Ginkgo leaf is the only herb included in this chapter that has not been used for over a thousand years. Its safety, therefore, is not 100 percent confirmed. Ginkgo is reported to be nontoxic, however, and millions of people are now using it. Its ultimate safety will only be known after several generations.

LIGUSTRUM

Pharmaceutical Name: Fructus Ligustri Lucidum
Treasures: *Yin jing*
Atmospheric Energy: Cool
Taste: Bitter and sweet
Organ Associations: Kidneys and Liver
Treasure Rating: ★★★★

Qualities Attributed to the Seed: Ligustrum is a very good *yin jing* tonic. Its action is very similar to that of Polygonum, except that it is a cool herb. It is used for all the same purposes as Polygonum, including blackening the hair or preventing premature graying. Thus it is considered to be an antiaging, rejuvenative herb. It strengthens the back and relieves soreness in the lower back and knees, and helps relieve aching in other joints. It is said to improve hearing and sharpen vision.

Ligustrum has gained quite a reputation in the past decade from the discovery that it has powerful immune-enhancing effects. In a study done in the United States, supported by the National Institutes of Health, it was found to prevent breakdown of the immune system when cancer patients were given chemotherapy and radiation therapy. Subsequent studies around the world have supported this action. It is now used clinically for this purpose in Japan and China.

Contraindications: Do not use when you have diarrhea due to cold. In cases of *yang* deficiency, it is often better to use Polygonum.

LONGAN

Pharmaceutical Name: Arillus Longan
Treasures: Blood and *qi*
Atmospheric Energy: Warm
Taste: Sweet
Organ Associations: Heart and Spleen
Treasure Rating: ★★★★

Qualities Attributed to the Aril: Longan is a wonderful and delicious tonic fruit used by the Chinese as a blood tonic, to build energy, to nurture the Heart, and to add luster and beauty to the skin. It is believed among the Chinese people that Longan is not only great for the skin but also a fantastic sex tonic for women. The most beautiful women in China have always eaten Longan. Longan is also beneficial to men. It is believed to have a calming effect and to add radiance to the skin and eyes.

Longan is often combined with other blood tonics such as Dang Gui and White Peony to build blood. It has a high organic iron content, about twenty times that of grapes and fifteen times that of spinach. Longan promotes peripheral circulation, warming up cold hands and feet.

It can be used to relieve heart palpitations, insomnia, forgetfulness, and anxiety associated with blood and *qi* deficiency and *shen* disturbance, especially when combined with *qi* tonics such as Ginseng, Codonopsis, and Astragalus and with *shen* tonics. Combined with *shen* tonics such as Ganoderma and Spirit Poria, it promotes tranquillity. This herb has been found to promote deep, refreshing sleep. For this purpose, it may be combined with Zizyphus. However, Longan itself is not a strong sedative. It is a fine *qi* tonic which increases physical stamina.

Contraindications: None, unless eaten in excess, in which case it may cause slight indigestion.

WHITE PEONY ROOT

Pharmaceutical Name: Radix Paeoniae Alba
Treasures: Blood
Atmospheric Energy: Slightly cold
Taste: Bitter and sour
Organ Associations: Liver and Spleen
Treasure Rating: ★★★★

Qualities Attributed to the Root: White Peony Root is a highly prized tonic herb used to build and cleanse the blood. It is one of the most highly regarded women's herbs used traditionally to help regulate the female hormonal cycle, to tonify and purify the blood, to help regulate menstruation, and to improve the quality of the skin. Men may use it as a blood tonic and blood cleanser as well. White Peony is commonly combined with Dang Gui, Prepared Rehmannia, Ligusticum, and other blood tonics.

It is also used to relax muscles, both striated and smooth. It is said to relieve cramps and spasms anywhere in the body. But in particular, it is considered to be very highly effective in relieving menstrual cramps as well as leg and foot cramps. White Peony contains an effective pain-reducing agent. It has a calming effect and is widely used as an emotional stabilizer, especially by women. When combined with Licorice Root, White Peony's antispasmodic and analgesic qualities are magnified. This combination is better than the sum of the parts.

White Peony Root is considered to be one of China's premium antiaging herbs and is very widely used to promote beauty. It purifies the blood, which in turn purifies the skin. There is an old Chinese saying that "a woman who consumes White Peony Root every day becomes as beautiful as the Peony flower itself." (The Peony is the national flower of China.) Women who use White Peony for an extended period of time find that their skin becomes finer, smoother, softer, and cleaner. The skin develops a soft radiance that looks young and alive. For beautiful skin, White Peony Root is usually combined with other antiaging, beauty-enhancing herbs such as Dang Gui, Pearl, Placenta, Schizandra, Astragalus, Royal Jelly, Asparagus Root, and Gynostemma.

Contraindications: Since the herb is cold, it should be used cautiously in cases of excess cold or deficiency of *yang*.

POLYGALA ROOT

Pharmaceutical Name: Radix Polygalae
Treasures: *Shen*
Atmospheric Energy: Slightly warm
Taste: Pungent and bitter
Organ Associations: Heart and Lungs
Treasure Rating: ★★★★½

Qualities Attributed to the Root: Polygala is one of the truly extraordinary tonic herbs in the entire Asian tonic herbal system. This herb first attained wide use in Daoist circles because it was believed to have powerful mind- and spirit-developing power. In fact, Polygala Root was believed to be an empowering substance in the class with wild Ginseng and Ganoderma. This root is traditionally used as a *shen* tonic to relax the mind, calm the emotions, and aid in the sleep process. However, it does not relax the mind in entirely the same manner as many *shen*-stabilizing herbs—Dragon Bone and Polygonum Stem, for example.

Many people claim that Polygala enhances dreaming and aids in creative thinking. And it aids not only creative thinking but the ability to manifest our ideas. In fact, the ancient name for this herb is the Will Strengthener. The herb is believed to have the ability to strengthen that part of the psyche we call the will. Daoists have long recommended using Polygala to strengthen the focus of the mind and to empower our thoughts so that they may be made real. The Daoists taught that our creative visualization, which they called *yi*, could be brought to reality by the will. Thus the will had to be strengthened. In fact, the will was virtually considered to be the fourth Treasure in what was otherwise called the Three Treasures system. Thus Polygala, as a will-strengthening herb, ranked high on the list of important herbs in the Daoist pharmacopoeia.

These days, Polygala may be used to strengthen the will of the spiritual seeker, or it may be used to strengthen the will of the more earthbound. It is used in formulations to build enough willpower to overcome obstacles and to achieve greater heights. For example, it can be used as the main ingredient in formulas to help stop smoking, or to break other habits, such as drug abuse, overeating, or compulsive behavior of any sort. Polygala has the unique power to provide the energy (the "power") to our will, so that we can overcome the obstacles that block us from becoming all that we can become. And it not only helps us break old, bad habits. It also helps strengthen our will to do new things, to achieve new heights—to start to work on a new project, to start exercising, to start and continue whatever we need to do to grow, to become a great human being. That is the magic of Polygala, the Will Strengthener.

Polygala has another quality that sets it apart from most other herbs, including the tonic herbs. It has the ability to connect the Kidney (sexual) energy with the Heart (love) energy. It does this by opening the energy flow between the Heart and Kidneys known as the Penetrating Vessel. The Penetrating Vessel is one of the energy channels that regulate the functions of the body-mind. It is called a psychic channel by the Daoists. Commonly, this vessel is blocked, resulting in a delinking of our sexual energy and our emotional feelings. It is essential for our true health and well-being that feelings of love and the functions of sex are united. Consuming Polygala for a period of time will have this result. The Will Strengthener thus has a unique power to deepen our experience and our feelings and to bring new levels of happiness into our lives.

Contraindications: Do not use excessively at first. Polygala Root is used to stabilize excessive dreaming, but in rare, extremely creative individuals, it may have a paradoxical reaction at first and actually increase the intensity of dreaming for a short period of time.

ZIZYPHUS SEED

Pharmaceutical Name: Semen Zizyphi Spinosae
Treasures: Blood and *shen*
Atmospheric Energy: Neutral
Taste: Sweet and sour
Organ Associations: Heart and Liver
Treasure Rating: ★★★½

Qualities Attributed to the Seed: Zizyphus is one of the most commonly used herbs in Chinese herbalism. It is an excellent tranquilizing herbal substance. It has been traditionally called Calm the Heart Seed. Being neutral in energy and mild in nature, it is the most commonly used lead herb in sedative formulas designed to help relax the mind and induce sound sleep. It is especially useful for people who are experiencing restless sleep with excessive, vivid dreams and/or nightmares.

It is categorized as a Heart-blood tonic, therefore directly calming the Heart, which is of course the seat of *shen* and determines our emotional stability. This is a very good herb for women who suffer insomnia due to a slight or profound anemic condition.

For simple, occasional insomnia due to stress or overthinking, Zizyphus may be brewed simply by itself, or it may be brewed as a tea with other *shen*-stabilizing herbs such as Polygonum Stem, Spirit Poria, and/or Ganoderma and consumed at bedtime.

Scientific research has demonstrated that Zizyphus Seed has antiarrhythmic activity in addition to its hypnotic and sedative effects.

Contraindications: Do not use when experiencing diarrhea. Zizyphus may cause drowsiness.

OTHER IMPORTANT TONICS AND SUPPORTIVE HERBS USED IN THE CHINESE TONIC HERBAL SYSTEM

Since most of the herbs used in Chinese herbalism are medicinal and fall into the inferior class, they do not fall in the scope of laymen's herbs. These must be prescribed by a doctor who is very familiar with them. However, besides the herbs previously described, there are another fifty or so that you will frequently come across when using the Chinese tonic herbs. Some of these are actually powerful tonics, almost in the same category as the above-described herbs. Others play supplemental roles. However, all of the following herbs are important.

White Atractylodes (★★★★) is a powerful *qi* tonic, almost in the same category of importance with other *qi* tonics such as Astragalus and Codonopsis. While rapidly and effectively building *qi*, White Atractylodes also invigorates the *yang* energy of the body, providing power and strength. In particular, it invigorates the *yang* energy of the Spleen, so that digestion is more efficient.

Hard physical activity performed while consuming White Atractylodes will result in muscle growth. It has a reputation as one of the primary herbs used by athletes to build powerful muscles and to provide endurance.

It is widely used to strengthen digestion and assimilation and to move moisture through the body. It is capable of regulating the appetite by increasing the appetite of those who are weak and by reducing appetite in those who are overzealous. In either case, White Atractylodes will help improve digestive efficiency. People with weak digestive systems will generally benefit greatly, and quickly, from this herb. It is useful for people who tend to experience diarrhea, bloating, abdominal pain, vomiting, and fatigue, especially during the summer or in hot climates.

White Atractylodes is especially useful for women who are low in *qi* and thus experience fatigue, digestive problems, and anemia.

Pharmacological and human clinical studies have shown that the herb has a diuretic action in patients with edema, but has little or no diuretic action in normal subjects. It has been shown in pharmacological studies to have mild hypoglycemic and liver-protective action.

Prepared Aconite (★★★) is a powerful herb that must be used moderately and with care. It has a hot energy and is tonic to *yang jing* and *qi*. It is one of the few commonly used tonic herbs that may have toxic qualities if used in too large quantities. Unprepared, raw Aconite is toxic. It is put through a special process to eliminate this toxicity. However, overuse of Prepared Aconite can result in overheating of the body. It is never used alone—it is always combined with other herbs.

Prepared Aconite is a powerful *yang* tonic used to rebuild Kidney *yang* when it has been depleted. Kidney *yang* deficiency is marked by chilliness, cold limbs, and impotence, infertility, frequent urination without pain, and some types of arthritis and rheumatism. Prepared Aconite is extraordinarily effective at waking up the *yang* energy, producing heat and warmth, and activating metabolism. It is also an extremely potent Kidney and bladder tonic and is effective at removing stagnant water due to coldness.

Aged Citrus (Tangerine) Peel (★) is a digestant. It has a warm and aromatic energy and affects the Spleen, stomach, and Lungs. It has a pungent and bitter taste. It falls into the classical category of *qi*-regulating herbs—that is, herbs that help *qi* move smoothly, preventing blockage, particularly in the digestive and respiratory systems. It is not a tonic herb but is often used in tonic formulations to improve their function. Sometimes strong *qi* formulas, in particular, can result in minor stagnation in the digestive tract if a *qi*-regulating herb is not included in the formula.

Aged Tangerine Peel is most commonly used to help eliminate digestive stagnation and to help relieve abdominal distension, belching, and bloating. It can be useful even if the stagnation reaches the extreme by resulting in nausea, diarrhea, and vomiting. Tangerine Peel is used to eliminate excess moisture in the digestive tract. It is often used in combination with *qi* tonics such as Ginseng, Codonopsis, and White Atractylodes to improve digestion and assimilation.

Because of its ability to eliminate dampness, Aged Tangerine Peel is often used to help eliminate phlegm, cough, and oppression in the lungs and to help clear the upper respiratory passages.

Albizzia Bark (★★★½) is used by the Chinese when one is experiencing emotional problems such as a broken heart or the experience of great loss. It has a neutral energy, is sweet-tasting, and affects the Heart and Liver. The bark of this exotic tree is an excellent *shen* stabilizer. It is calming and improves mood. It helps with anxiety, insomnia, irritability, anger, forgetfulness, excessive worry. It is commonly used for any chronic emotional upsets.

Albizzia Flower (★★★★½) is even better than the bark. It has the same *shen*-stabilizing ability as the bark but has much stronger *shen*-lifting (mood-elevating) ability. It is one of the best herbs to use for people who are severely depressed, very angry, despondent, or paranoid. I have used the flower successfully for numerous cases of broken heart and despair. This is one of the ultimate *shen* tonic herbs.

Achyranthes Root (★★) is frequently used in *yang* tonic formulations. It is a mild *jing* tonic. Its main function generally revolves around its ability to guide other herbs to the Kidneys, genitals, and legs.

Alisma (★½) is a commonly used herb in Chinese herbalism. It helps strengthen water metabolism, which is a critical body function. Alisma has a cold energy, is mildly sweet, and affects the Kidney and bladder functions. It rids the body of excess dampness through the urinary tract. It is mild and safe, with mild tonic qualities, especially to the Kidneys and bladder, and to the Spleen and stomach as well. It is an excellent herb to use in a tonic program by those who need to stimulate fluid function, so long as you do not have a cold constitution.

Alisma is used in medicinal herbalism to treat damp-heat conditions, which means conditions that are associated with chronic or acute infections. It is one of the primary herbs used to treat such conditions associated with the Kidney and bladder systems, such as leukorrhea, where the discharge is yellow, or urinary tract infections. It is also used to treat conditions such as lung congestion where the phlegm is tinged yellow or green. It is often used for obesity, especially for people who carry a lot of water weight and tend to have rosy complexions. It is also commonly used by people who have difficulty urinating and by diabetics. It is used routinely by older men to help cleanse the prostate gland and improve urinary function. If you are experiencing a medical condition that you think involves an infection, see a doctor immediately. Urinary tract infections can be serious and can spread quickly to internal organs. Don't take a chance. However, you can use Alisma along with most antibiotics, since it is a very safe herb. This is a common practice in Japan and China. It can be used in large quantities. In fact, it usually requires fairly large doses to do its best work.

Amber (★★★½) is primarily used in Chinese herbalism to relax the nerves and calm the mind. It is safe and effective as a mild tranquilizer. It has a neutral energy, is sweet, and affects the Heart and Liver functions. It is believed that by calming the mind by consuming Amber and other *shen*-stabilizing agents, the mind has the opportunity to rest, regain strength and focus.

Amber is thus used in formulas both for calming anxiety and for improving the power of the mind. It is believed to improve concentration, memory, and alertness when consumed in moderation over a continuous period of time, especially when combined with other mind-strengthening tonics such as Schizandra, Lycium, Polygonatum sibericum, Deer Antler, Ginseng, Gynostemma, and Acanthopanax, and along with other *shen* stabilizers such as Biota, Polygonum Stem, and Zizyphus. Amber is always used with other herbs in a formulation.

Amber has excellent effects for people experiencing palpitations due to anxiety, insomnia, excessive dreaming, and nightmares. Amber can be especially beneficial to those who suffer excess tension due to stress.

Donkey Skin Glue (★★★★) is a powerful blood and *yin* tonic routinely used in Chinese herbalism, especially in women's formulas. The fried Skin of the donkey has a neutral energy, a sweet taste, and affects the Lungs, Liver, and Kidneys. It is commonly combined with other major tonic herbs to fortify the entire body after illness, injury, or surgery. It can be used by anyone suffering from blood deficiency. It is usually combined with Ginseng, Astragalus, Dang Gui, and Prepared Rehmannia.

It may be combined with herbs that have a hemostatic action (they stop bleeding). However, since bleeding is serious, a doctor's supervision is required.

Donkey Skin Glue has *yin* properties that are useful in *yin* deficiency syndrome, manifesting as dry cough, dry mouth, and irritability. It may be combined with other *yin* herbs such as American Ginseng, Glehnia, Ophiopogon, and Asparagus Root to replenish fluids.

Biota Seed (★★★½) is most commonly used in Chinese tonic herbalism as a component in *shen* tonic formulations. It has a neutral energy, a sweet taste, and affects the Heart and Kidneys.

It is calming and sedative. It can be used to help allay fear, anxiety, and insomnia. When combined with Zizyphus, Schizandra, and Poria, Biota is believed to be nourishing to the Heart. Because of the oily nature of the herb, it can help with constipation.

Cinnamon Bark (★★★★) is one of the most warming of all herbs. It has a hot energy, a pungent and sweet taste, and affects the Kidneys, Heart, and Liver. It is a strong *yang* tonic which may be used to correct Kidney *yang* deficiency, which will generally present itself by an aversion to cold, cold hands and feet, weak kidneys, backache, and lack of sexual energy. It is usually combined with *yin* and *yang jing* tonic herbs and with *qi* tonics to build energy and to fire up sexual energy.

Cinnamon Bark promotes good circulation and enables *qi* to circulate freely. It has a hot energy which warms the body at its core. Cinnamon Bark is used to warm up cold visceral organs and to calm the nerves. However, its energy is said to "move upward and float." In moving upward, it disperses energy blocks in the neck and shoulders and thus relieves tension in this area. In moving outward ("floating"), it warms the flesh. Prolonged use is said to result in a more youthful, rosy-cheeked complexion and will help clear the skin of blemishes. It is also used medicinally to treat headaches, abdominal pain (especially when combined with Licorice Root), and to promote menstruation.

Cinnamon Bark also generates *qi* and blood, especially when combined with *qi* and blood tonics such as Astragalus. Use with Dang Gui for menstrual pain due to poor circulation.

Cinnamon Twig (no stars), the young cinnamon branch, strengthens the body and is said to result in a more youthful complexion. Cinnamon Twig can be used to relax neck and shoulder tension. It is categorized as a warm herb, capable of warming the entire body, and is primarily used in Chinese herbalism to open blood channels and thus to improve circulation. However, Cinnamon Twig lacks the deep *yang*-tonifying effect of the aged bark.

Cistanches (★★★★) is one of the more popular, and more potent, *yang* tonic herbs and is found in many formulas designed to strengthen sexual function, treat impotence, and strengthen the back and knees. It has a warm energy, a sweet and salty taste, and affects the Kidneys and large intestine. It is used not only in men's sexual formulas but also in women's, particularly to increase fertility.

It is widely reported by men who have taken Cistanches for more than a few weeks that their sexual prowess has increased noticeably. The highly regarded tenth-century imperial manual on health and sexual conduct, *The Essence of Medical Prescriptions*, compiled by a Chinese physician living in Japan by the name of Tamba Yasuyori, described numerous formulations that would enhance male potency. Cistanches was included in 80 percent of these formulas. The ancient classics indicate that Cistanches increases both the flow of *yang* energy and blood to the genitals.

Youthfulness is very much associated with sexual vigor, whether one uses this sexual vigor sexually or converts the energy to other creative outlets. When the Kidney *yin* and *yang* are strong, a person can flourish. He or she will be full of energy, high in spirit, creative, and strong-minded and will appear radiantly healthy and attractive to others.

Cistanches has a secondary benefit, in that it improves the function of the bowels, resulting in healthy bowel movements. This is a result of increased *qi* in the large intestine.

Cnidium Seed (★★★½) has been commonly used in formulations designed to warm the Kidneys and strengthen *yang* energy. It has a warm energy, is pungent and bitter-tasting, and affects the Kidneys and Spleen. It is primarily used for overcoming sexual malaise and strengthening sexual potency. The classics repeatedly mention it as an aphrodisiac. It was used almost routinely in imperial formulas designed specifically for the emperor. Cnidium Seed was often used in combination with Cuscuta Seed in aphrodisiac formulations, since the two herbs are believed to work synergistically, enhancing one another. It is also used to increase fertility in both men and women. Cnidium has some astringent quality, which means that it will help prevent premature ejaculation in men. Furthermore, Cnidium Seed has disinfectant qualities and may be used externally as a wash on sores, particularly in the genital region.

Coix (★★★), also known as Job's Tears, is a food-herb that many people confuse with barley. It has a cold energy and a bland or slightly sweet taste. It is used as a general health tonic, primarily benefiting the functions of the Spleen, Lungs, and skin. It improves the flow of water throughout the body, so it can be used by those who are experiencing water stagnancy, abdominal bloating, and edema (excessive water weight). Puffed Coix (just like puffed oats, corn, or wheat—"shot out of cannons!") is beneficial to those who suffer from loose stool or diarrhea. Coix is also commonly used in many formulas in Asia for arthritis and rheumatism, since these conditions are associated with "excess moisture."

Coix is considered to be beneficial to the skin, in terms of both beauty and health. Combined with herbs like White Peony and Dang Gui, it is very nourishing to the skin. It is said that by using Coix, one's skin becomes especially smooth and soft. Coix is used in Asia to eliminate coarse skin. Coix has long been believed to be capable of helping to reduce moles and to eliminate warts and other blemishes. Recent research conducted in Japan has demonstrated that raw Coix contains an antitumor agent that, in large doses, may be useful in the treatment of cancer, and in particular cancer of the skin. Coix has also been shown to have antiviral activity.

Cornus (★★★½) is a mild *yin* tonic that acts upon the Kidneys, most specifically upon the urogenital system. It has a warm energy and a very sour taste. Its tonic action is highly magnified by its powerful astringent action. When combined with other tonic herbs, Cornus becomes a powerhouse and makes the other herbs much more powerful as well. Being a warm *yin* tonic makes it a somewhat unusual herb. Its great power does not lie in the actual amount of *yin* provided by the Cornus itself—it lies in Cornus' astringent action on the urogenital organs.

Cornus is very sour, and like all sour herbs, it helps control ejaculation of sperm and helps treat impotence, premature ejaculation, and frequent urination due to weak bladder. Because of its warm nature and because of its direct action on the genital function, many Asian herbalists consider Cornus to have aphrodisiac qualities. Like all true Kidney tonics, Cornus helps strengthen the back and knees, clears the mind, and improves hearing. It is well known for its benefits for people experiencing dizziness. Those who are deficient in *yin jing* can combine Cornus with *yin* herbs. Those who are deficient in *yang jing* can combine Cornus with *yang* herbs. In either case, Cornus will strengthen *jing* by conserving it.

A quinol glucoside that acts as a urinary antiseptic has been isolated in Cornus. Extracts have shown antibacterial activity against *Staphylococcus aureus, Salmonella typhula*, and *Shigella dysenteriae*. Extracts have also shown antiallergenic effects. Cornus will help reduce perspiration in those who sweat due to illness, weakness, or fear. Mixed with the appropriate herbs, Cornus is very useful for stabilizing excessive or prolonged menstrual bleeding due to deficiency and weakness.

Crataegus Fruit (★) strengthens digestion. It helps to remove stagnated food from the digestive tract and to restore normal functioning of the Spleen, stomach, and Liver in digesting, transporting, and distributing nutrients. It is slightly warm and has a sour and sweet taste. Crataegus, also known as

Hawthorn Berry, is commonly used to relieve indigestion that has resulted in abdominal distension, belching, acid regurgitation, stuffiness, anorexia, abdominal pain, nausea, vomiting, and irregular bowel movements (diarrhea or constipation). In China, Crataegus is often consumed as the main ingredient in a tea, or combined with a couple of other digestive herbs, when one has consumed too much meat or greasy food. Crataegus is excellent at digesting these.

Crataegus has become an extremely popular herb in Europe because of its beneficial influence on hypertension, hyperlipemia (high blood fat), and high cholesterol. Often the leaf extract is used. Crataegus can be used to treat symptoms of coronary heart disease, especially when combined with herbs that improve circulation, such as Salvia, Notoginseng, Ginkgo, and Ligusticum.

Cuscuta Seed (★★★½) is commonly used in tonic formulations designed to benefit *yin* and *yang jing*. It has a neutral energy, a pungent and sweet taste, and affects the Kidney and Liver functions. It is most commonly used to strengthen the urogenital functions. It is used to treat impotence, premature ejaculation, frequent urination, and leukorrhea as well as tinnitus and aching lower back, symptoms that often accompany deficient Kidney conditions that can cause sexual weakness.

Cuscuta Seed gently but efficiently helps tonify both *yin* and *yang*. People suffering from Kidney *yin* deficiency will tend to experience dizziness, blurred vision, spots in front of the eyes, and ringing in the ears. Habitual consumption of Cuscuta can improve vision and clear away these symptoms.

Cuscuta will build *yin* Essence (*yin jing*) and is thus considered to be an antiaging herb. It is used to build sperm, increase fertility in both men and women, and is listed as an aphrodisiac in all traditional Chinese pharmacopoeias.

Cuscuta will be used with either *yin* or *yang* tonic herbs depending on the specifics of the person's condition. It is almost always combined with Cnidium Seed because the two enhance each other. Cuscuta Seed helps consolidate the Essence (*yin jing*) and thus slows down aging and prevents loss of body fluids. This type of herb is critical in any program designed to rejuvenate the body and prolong life.

Dragon Bone (★★★½) is a *shen*-stabilizing substance. It has a neutral energy, is sweet and astringent, and enters the Heart, Liver, Kidneys, and large intestine. It calms the Liver and suppresses hyperactivity of Liver *yang*. This results in a strong calming effect, which can be described as both sedating and relaxing. Dragon Bone is one of the primary natural substances known for calming excitability and palpitation.

Dragon Bone can be used as an effective astringent herb. It is often used in formulas to control seminal emission, leukorrhagia, frequent urination, chronic diarrhea, excessive perspiration due to weakness, and excessive uterine bleeding. It is often found in formulas designed to enhance male sexual performance. In this usage, it has a calming effect on the mind, preventing premature ejaculation, as well as the astringent action, which literally locks in the semen.

Dragon Bone is a wonderful supplement for those who suffer from insomnia, restlessness, apprehension, palpitations, anxiety, irritability, anger, frustration, tension, fear, or any of the symptoms that require an astringent. Dragon Bone changes people's lives. And it is extremely safe.

Poria (★★★★) has traditionally been used in Chinese herbalism as a *qi* tonic to benefit the internal organs. It is a solid fungus which grows on the roots of old pine trees. The *Spirit Farmer's Pharmacopoeia* said that "Poria is tranquilizing to the mind, and long-term taking of Poria can relieve hunger and lengthen the life." It is one of the primary longevity herbs and is included in most longevity tonics. Poria is also mildly sedative and is widely used as an antistress herb.

It is a mild, safe, and effective diuretic. It has a neutral energy, a bland taste, and affects the Heart, Spleen, and Kidney functions. Poria is used in hundreds of classical formulas to improve the flow of water through the body. It is especially used in *qi* tonics for this purpose.

Recent research has discovered that Poria is a powerful immune system tonic. It has been found to induce the production in human beings of alpha-interferon. It is common in Chinese and Japanese formulas used to build the immune systems of cancer patients.

Spirit Poria (★★★★½) is a very good *shen* tonic herb. It has a neutral energy, is bland or very mildly sweet, and affects the Heart, Spleen, and Kidney functions. It is primarily the same herb as Poria, except that it is the center of the mushroom, where the root of the host wood runs. The pine root is allowed to remain and represents about 20 percent of each slice of Spirit Poria. The chemistry and the energy of the wood have been changed by the fungus. Spirit Poria was used by Daoists and has been held in the highest esteem by spiritual seekers. It is believed by the Daoists to have a very special power to lift *shen* and to help develop the Spirit. It is one of the major *shen* tonics and *shen*-stabilizing substances and has acquired a special reputation for its overall emotional balancing benefits. By stabilizing the emotions, the true mind is able to develop fully, unhindered by emotional distraction. Unlike Biota and Zizyphus, it is drying and can be used by people who suffer from fluid stagnation.

Besides these *shen* actions, Spirit Poria still has the same actions as regular Poria with regard to its ability to move water and tonify the immune functions.

Gastrodia (½ ★) is one of the most precious of the medicinal herbs used in Chinese herbalism. It has a neutral energy, a sweet taste, and affects the Liver function. It is primarily used to counter the symptoms caused by "endogenous wind," which manifests in such conditions as childhood convulsions, convulsions resulting from high fever, headaches, and epilepsy induced by fright. Gastrodia is commonly used to treat spasms in the legs, abdomen, feet, and back.

It is the main herb in formulas used to treat childhood convulsions. Because there are different causes of childhood convulsions, a medical practitioner should select the herbs that are combined with the Gastrodia. It is rarely used alone. It is combined in sophisticated formulas designed to treat each specific problem.

Gastrodia is also the main herb used in Chinese herbalism to treat headaches. The Chinese describe at least four primary headache syndromes, with many subtle variations, for which Gastrodia is effective. These are: (1) headaches caused by hyperactivity of Liver *yang*, (2) headaches caused by upward movement of wind-phlegm, (3) headaches caused by deficiency of blood and *yin*, and (4) chronic headaches and migraines.

Gastrodia is used to treat chronic dizziness and vertigo. These, too, are "endogenous wind" conditions. It is also used in formulas to treat wind stroke, hemiplegia, and numbness of the limbs. In China, it has been used to treat tetanus, but if you step on a rusty nail, hurry to a doctor and get a tetanus shot.

In addition, Gastrodia is beneficial for preventing premature graying and loss of the hair. It improves circulation in the scalp and, when combined with Polygonum, stimulates circulation in the follicles and promotes the health of the hair. It is therefore used both internally and externally as a hair tonic.

Gecko (★★★★½) is used to tonify the Lung and Kidney functions. It is extremely effective and is very highly prized as a tonic. The part used is the tail of the lizard. It has a neutral energy, a salty taste, and is tonic to the Kidney and Liver functions. It is the lead herb in many patent formulations and is regarded to be in the same league as Deer Antler and Cordyceps as a *yang* tonic to the Kidneys. Like Cordyceps, it builds both *yang* and *yin* and is therefore considered highly nourishing. It is also considered to be an excellent blood and *yin jing* tonic.

Gecko is commonly used in men's sexual-potency-enhancing tonic formulations. Taken consistently for a period of time, Gecko is extremely reliable as a tonic to the male sexual functions. Though it is not considered aphrodisiac, it does have long-lasting results once they kick in, somewhere between a week and a month after you start taking it. Like all *yang* Kidney tonics, Gecko strengthens the lower back.

Gecko is a powerful Lung tonic. It is traditionally used in a great many Lung tonic formulations, as it is said to enhance the extraction of *qi* from the air. Used with Ginseng and/or Astragalus, it empowers breathing and builds endurance. No more powerful energy-building combination exists in Chinese tonic herbalism. That is why Gecko formulas have always been a favorite of Chinese gung fu masters and are now a favorite of athletes around the world. Gecko is also used for coughs due to cold and to relieve asthma that is stimulated by cold.

Polyrachis (★★★★★) is a genus of large ant indigenous to various mountain regions of China. Polyrachis tonics are now widely consumed in Asia to promote strength and sexual vigor and as a powerful antiaging agent. Extensive research has proven that Polyrachis is highly nutritious and has powerful medicinal effects. Polyrachis is considered a premium adaptogenic substance in the same ranks as Ginseng, Acanthopanax, Schizandra, Cordyceps, Astragalus, Ganoderma, and Gynostemma, the superstars of Chinese tonic herbalism.

Polyrachis is widely used to boost the immune system, or to maintain already strong immune functions. It has been established to have double-direction benefits on the immune system, so it is used by anyone with any immune disorder to regulate immune functions.

Polyrachis is widely believed to prevent common symptoms associated with aging, such as lumbago, memory loss, joint problems, fatigue, climacteric symptoms, cardiovascular disease, and so on. Polyrachis strengthens the entire Kidney system, including the sexual functions, skeletal structures, and renal system. It also strengthens the nervous system, digestive functions, detoxification functions, and muscular system. Polyrachis products, therefore, have become extremely popular with middle-aged and elderly consumers in Asia. Polyrachis is called the "forever young" nutritional supplement.

Young people in China seem to be major advocates of Polyrachis as well. Young men and women use it to increase energy on a daily as well as long-term basis. Students in particular have made Polyrachis elixirs a virtual craze in cities like Shanghai, Hong Kong, and Beijing. It is commonly used by those who have become fatigued or exhausted due to excess workloads or other forms of stress, including mental sources. Polyrachis is noticeably energizing when consumed for a short period of time and builds long-term energy if used continuously.

These ants can carry a load 100 times their own weight, and people have long felt that consuming the nontoxic varieties of Polyrachis can increase physical and mental strength. Because of its long- and short-term energy-boosting qualities, Polyrachis tonics are becoming popular as preworkout elixirs in Hong Kong and Taiwan, where many adults visit health clubs regularly. Polyrachis is ideal for athletes, especially when combined with Ginseng, Acanthopanax, and other similar tonics.

Dried Ginger ($\frac{1}{2}$★) is used in Chinese herbalism primarily to warm up the stomach and Spleen and thus to improve digestion and relieve cold conditions associated with these organs, which generally cause poor digestion. It has a hot energy, a spicy flavor, and affects the Spleen, Kidney, Heart, and Lung functions. Thus when it is combined with a Kidney *yang* herb, it will provide heat to the Kidneys. The herb itself has only very minor tonic effects, but it tends to magnify the tonic qualities of other herbs, particularly *qi* tonics like Ginseng and Astragalus.

Fresh Ginger is sometimes used in Chinese herbalism as well. It is called *shangjiang*. It is used for just the opposite conditions: dryness and heat. It moistens and cools the interior.

Glehnia (★★★½) is a very good moistening tonic. It clears the lungs and tonifies *yin*. Glehnia is cold and sweet and affects the Lungs and stomach. It is the perfect herb to use when the lungs are dry due to smoking, smog, dry or dusty air, or excessive talking or singing. It can also be used to treat common dry chronic cough and hoarseness. If such a condition persists, see your health practitioner.

Glehnia helps replenish body fluids. It is a very useful herb in dry climates or during dry weather. It can also be used to replenish fluids during and after an illness or surgery. People who are chronically dehydrated will find this herb a lifesaver. It is a great component of a homemade sports drink.

Sea Horse and *Sea Dragon* (★★★★) are closely related species of fish that are used in Chinese tonic herbal formulations. They are both considered to be powerful *yang* tonics and are especially renowned as potent sexual tonics, especially in men's formulations. Sea Horse is slightly weaker than Sea Dragon. They have a warm energy, salty taste, and affect the Kidney functions. They provide *yang* to the Kidneys and have a reputation as reliable aphrodisiacs.

Jujube Date (★★★½) is a commonly used herb, especially in formulas that use Ginseng. It is warm and sweet and affects the Spleen and stomach. It is the classic sidekick to Ginseng. Anytime you use Ginseng, you can use Jujube. The date is believed to enhance the activity of Ginseng while smoothing out any rough edges the Ginseng may have. It harmonizes the ingredients in a formula, making the whole formula smooth in both taste and action. However, it is much more than just an adjunctive herb. It provides excellent energy and is a powerful *qi* tonic in its own right.

It helps the Spleen and stomach extract the energy from food and drink at maximum efficiency. It is also an excellent blood tonic. Jujube also has an emotionally calming effect. It is a mild *shen* stabilizer.

Ligusticum (★★★½) is one of the primary blood-vitalizing herbs used in Chinese herbalism. Blood-vitalizing herbs improve circulation. It has a warm energy, a pungent and bitter flavor, and affects the Liver and Heart functions. It is very widely used in treating menstrual disorders because it is so effective at activating blood flow and relieving pain associated with blood and *qi* stagnation. It warms the uterus and decongests swelling in the pelvic basin. In addition to its blood-*vitalizing* effects, Ligusticum is a good blood tonic.

Though it was not classically recognized as a major Heart tonic, Ligusticum has recently been recognized as being beneficial to the heart muscle and circulatory system. Its action in this regard is similar to that of Notoginseng and Salvia. It significantly enhances myocardial circulation and is now being widely used clinically in China to treat and prevent heart disease. Ligusticum is related to Dang Gui, and they share some of the same characteristics. They also share some components. However, Dang Gui is a stronger blood tonic and Ligusticum is a stronger blood vitalizer and analgesic.

Ligusticum is also widely used to relieve the pain associated with rheumatism and arthritis and in formulations to treat colds, flus, sinus congestion, and various skin disorders.

Lily Bulb (★★½) is primarily used to moisten the Lungs. It has a slightly cool energy, is sweet, and affects the Lungs and Heart. It is very effective at relieving dry cough and dry throat. It thus is excellent for smokers, singers, public speakers, fire-eaters, and those who use their voices excessively for any reason.

Lily Bulb has mild but effective influence on the emotions. It is capable of calming agitation and relieving anxiety, grief, and despair. In this regard, however, it is weaker than Lily Flower.

Lily Flower (★★★½). The Chinese call Lily "the plant for forgetting care and sorrow." They believe that by eating or drinking a tea of Lily Flower, one is able to forget unpleasant memories and sorrow. Lily Flower is high in iron and builds blood, and also contains several vitamins.

Male Silk Moth (★★★★½) has a long history in China of being used as a male sex tonic. It is warm, has a salty and pungent taste, and affects the Kidney and Liver functions. Rich in protein, cephalin, and male hormones, Male Silk Moth is conducive to the normal growth of the body and the formation and evolution of the male reproductive organs. It is used to nourish the Kidneys, accelerate the growth of sperm and marrow, and stimulate the nervous system. Male Silk Moth is considered in Asia to be an extremely potent male sexual stimulant and tonic.

Even though silkworms are abundant in China, the moth that can be used for this tonic is rare. The male silk moths must be separated one by one from the females. Only the male moth is used as an herb because it is the male sexual hormones that are desired. Within minutes of escaping from the cocoon, the male moths are separated from the females. This must be done before the moths have an opportunity to copulate. Once the male moth has copulated, it is no longer useful as a sex hormone donor. The male moth is then dried or preserved in alcohol.

Male Silk Moth tonic formulations are universally powerful. The moth extract is usually mixed with other powerful Kidney *yang* tonics such as Deer Antler, Gecko, Cordyceps, Morinda, and Epimedium and with *qi* tonics such as Ginseng, Astragalus, and Acanthopanax. Male Silk Moth is rarely available in America in bulk form, but a number of products are available which are extremely interesting.

Fresh Rehmannia (★★½) is used in formulas that require the *yin*-tonifying benefits of Rehmannia but also require a cooling or anti-inflammatory effect. Fresh Rehmannia is often used in cases where a person is experiencing such warming symptoms as hot flashes. It is used less commonly than Prepared Rehmannia in tonic herbalism but can be very useful in cases of *yin* deficiency.

Ophiopogon Root (★★★★½) is very similar in its actions to wild Asparagus Root, a close relative. It has a cold energy, is sweet and bitter, and affects the Lungs, Heart, and stomach. It is primarily used as a *yin* tonic, and especially as a *yin* tonic to the Heart and Lungs. It is excellent for moistening any dryness in the body. Being a cold herb, it can cool down hot symptoms and relieve *yin* deficiency conditions such as *yin* deficiency insomnia and irritability, especially when blended with herbs such as fresh Rehmannia and Asparagus Root.

It is a great herb for people who experience hot, dry lungs. Smokers and people exposed to smoke, smog, desert heat, and dust will benefit from a daily dose of this herb. Singers and public speakers will find that Ophiopogon moistens the throat and vocal cords, improving vocal quality. It helps relieve sticky sputum. For dry throat and lungs, Ophiopogon can be combined with herbs such as Asparagus Root, Glehnia, and fresh Rehmannia.

The Daoists perceived an even deeper level of purpose for consuming this herb. They considered Ophiopogon a major *shen* tonic herb. Like Asparagus Root, it was considered extremely valuable for mastering one's own Heart. It is found in a wide number of Daoist formulas. By cooling down the heat in the Heart, it helps to steady the emotions and control the mind. Combine with major *shen*-developing tonics such as wild Ginseng, Ganoderma, and Asparagus Root.

Polygonatum Sibericum (★★★★) is used as a *yin* and *qi* tonic and is said to have a specific benefit on the energy of the Heart and brain. It has a neutral energy and sweet taste. It affects the Kidney, Heart, Spleen, and Lung functions. It is used in *shen* and *jing* tonics to nourish the brain and strengthen the mind. Polygonatum is believed to be restorative to mental vitality, especially when the mind has been overworked, overstressed, or is in a state of exhaustion. It is not a stimulant and thus does not have instant effects. However, taken over a relatively short period of time (a week to a month), this herb is a potent mind tonic. Its effects are long-lasting. And if consumed regularly, Polygonatum can prevent mental and emotional breakdown when you are experiencing heavy mental loads. Regular use sharpens memory, concentration, wakefulness, and focus. It is a great herb for students, executives, airplane pilots, emergency room personnel, and so on.

It can be combined with Panax Ginseng, Siberian Ginseng (Acanthopanax), Deer Antler, Ganoderma, Walnut, Ginkgo Leaf, Schizandra, Lycium, Ant, Gynostemma, and various *shen* tonics such as Asparagus Root, Spirit Poria, and Pearl for a super brain tonic.

For people with weak digestion (deficient Spleen), the herb may be mixed with Astragalus, White Atractylodes, Poria, and Codonopsis. These herbs may be added to the above-mentioned formulas to improve digestion of the formulas.

Polygonum Stem (★★★), the stem of its more famous root, is a powerful *shen*-stabilizing agent used in many formulas to calm the Spirit, steady the mind, and promote sound sleep. It has a neutral energy, sweet taste, and affects the Heart and Liver. It has a smooth action and is very safe to use. It is generally combined with other *shen*-stabilizing herbs such as Zizyphus Seed, Biota,

Dragon Bone, Oyster Shell, and Spirit Poria, and with other Heart-blood tonics such as Longan to treat insomnia due to Heart-blood deficiency. Such insomnia is characterized by difficulty in falling asleep, as opposed to insomnia due to Heart *yin* deficiency, which is characterized by difficulty *staying* asleep.

Prince Ginseng (★★★½) is an excellent *qi* tonic that is often substituted for Ginseng. It has a neutral energy, a sweet and slightly bitter taste, and affects the Spleen and Lungs. Being *yin*, it can be used much as American Ginseng is used. As a *qi* tonic, it can be combined with Dioscorea and other *qi* tonics to tonify *qi* while not creating excess heat. As a *yin* tonic, it can be combined with Glehnia, Dendrobium, Polygonatum, and/or Ophiopogon to nourish the Lungs. Used with these herbs, it can generate fluids and allay thirst. With the same herbs, and with the addition of Fritillaria, it is excellent for dry coughing and difficult breathing. Used with Hemp Seed, Cistanches, Dang Gui, and/or Polygonum, it can help relieve constipation.

Traditionally, Prince Ginseng has been considered to be a good mild substitute for Ginseng, especially American Ginseng. However, it is a different kind of herb—it does not contain ginsenosides. Some people are now using Prince Ginseng *and* American Ginseng in the same formula.

Pueraria Root (½★) is among the most important of the medicinal herbs used in Chinese herbalism. It is very widely used. It has a cool energy, a pungent and sweet taste, and affects the Spleen and stomach. It is particularly important in the treatment of many common ailments, from headaches and stiff shoulders to fevers and the common cold. It is an herb that everyone familiar with Chinese herbs uses from time to time. Chinese doctors use it daily. In tonic herbalism, it is only used on the rare occasions when one is suffering a minor ailment for which Pueraria Root is helpful.

It belongs to a class of herbs that are said to "release the exterior." It helps to open the pores at the surface of the body and is therefore excellent for relieving fevers accompanying colds. It is commonly combined with Ephedra, Cinnamon Twig, White Peony, and fresh Ginger to relieve the symptoms associated with the common cold. These are warm herbs. This combination is used when a person is experiencing stiffness and pain in the upper back and/or neck, headache, aversion to wind and cold, and fever.

If a person is experiencing heat symptoms such as fever, headache, and red painful eyes and dry throat, then Pueraria will be combined with cooling herbs such as Bupleurum and Scutellaria.

If you are ill, it is best to see a health practitioner. But Pueraria is an extremely useful herb once you have learned the basics of Chinese herbalism.

Salvia (★) is not a tonic herb because it does not nourish any of the Three Treasures. However, it is a very important herb in the tonic health system because of its critical adjunctive role as a circulation enhancer. It is used in much the same manner as raw Notoginseng, except that Salvia is a cooling herb which can dispel heat. As a cooling herb, it can be used to treat problems where there is blood stagnation (areas where blood flow is sluggish) or blood stasis (areas where blood flow is entirely blocked or impeded) accompanied by heat, as is the case in heart disease and skin eruptions. Salvia has a bitter taste and affects the Heart function.

It is perhaps the primary herb now used in Chinese herbalism to prevent and treat heart disease, including angina pectoris. Salvia can be combined with Ligusticum and Notoginseng to improve circulation in the myocardium, or it can be used alone. It is now believed in China to have preventive action.

It is one of the primary herbs used to treat hot skin diseases, including acne and boils. Such sores are hot (inflamed and red) and stagnant. Salvia is used to clear them out and cool the area down. Salvia can be used with Dang Gui, Pearl, White Peony, and Scutellaria to help clear the skin.

It is also extremely valuable for treating menstrual problems, including irregular, absent, or painful menstruation. For this purpose, it would be combined with some of the following herbs: Dang Gui, Ligusticum, Carthamus, Moutan, Red Peony, Achyranthes, and White Peony.

Royal Jelly (★★★★½) is a popular natural food substance produced by worker bees for their queen. This incredibly nutritious whole food is rich in a very broad spectrum of important vitamins, minerals, and other substances essential to radiant health. Royal Jelly is believed to be an important cosmetic aid and is said to beautify the skin, eyes, and hair. It is available in many commercially prepared products or can be obtained fresh, straight from the hive. It is often combined with supertonic herbs such as Ginseng, Dang Gui, and Schizandra.

Placenta (★★★★★), because of its role in nurturing new life, is considered to be the most profound substance for replenishing *yin* and *yang jing* and blood. It is also considered to be a major *qi* tonic. It is the dominant ingredient in many of the greatest restorative formulations, where quick and powerful replenishment is required. It regulates hormonal balance and prevents degeneration. Though strange to many westerners, it is widely used in Asia.

Polyporus (★★½), a woody mushroom similar to Ganoderma, is a *qi* tonic used to improve kidney and bladder functions. Recent research conducted in Japan may indicate that Polyporus is a potent immune system potentiator, similar in this regard to Ganoderma.

Lohanguo (★★½) is a very sweet fruit. It is used to relieve lung congestion and to cool the lungs, thus "clearing heat" such as one might experience on a hot, smoggy day. As a Lung tonic, this herb also helps benefit energy and the skin.

Walnut Kernel (★★★½) is considered to be a useful and important Essence tonic with both *yin* and *yang* energies. It is said to tonify the functions of the Kidneys and Liver and thus by Chinese reckoning is useful as a sexual tonic. It is also used as a brain tonic to strengthen the mind. Walnuts, because of their lubricating qualities, are said to beautify the skin and to improve the functioning of the colon. They are usually combined with Longan fruit. The skin of the Walnut is considered to be bitter and slightly toxic, so for culinary and tonic purposes, the best organic walnuts are peeled.

Ephedra (no stars) is truly a remarkable herb, simultaneously one of the most wonderful and yet most controversial natural substances being used in herbalism today. Ephedra ranks up with Ginseng in importance in Chinese herbalism, but it is not a tonic herb and is therefore not tonic to any of the Three Treasures. It has a warm energy and a spicy taste. It affects primarily the Lungs. Because it is a medicinal herb with potential for side effects, it must be used properly and carefully to be safe and effective. Ephedra has substantial therapeutic value for a wide range of disorders, many of which are well understood scientifically. But it also has the potential to be abused and misused, and that has resulted in the controversial marketing and use of Ephedra as a diet (weight-reducing) herb in the United States over the last few years.

Ephedra, which is widely known by its Chinese name of Ma Huang, is an extremely versatile herb in the hands of a professional, knowledgeable herbalist. Ma Huang is a powerful diaphoretic and decongestant. It can be used, and is used, for many common disorders including the common cold, influenza, sinus problems, headaches, fevers, edema, arthritis, and rheumatism. Ma Huang is used in Chinese herbalism for chronic lung disorders such as asthma and bronchitis. As a diaphoretic, it causes perspiration and is therefore said to "relieve the surface."

Ma Huang is a powerful thermogenic agent—that is, it increases the burning of calories in the body by stimulating special tissue known as brown fat, which in turn stimulates the burning of the much more abundant white fat that is the bane of so many Americans.

Thermogenic studies showed that when Ma Huang is combined with caffeine and aspirin, or aspirin analogues, its effects are greatly enhanced in the fight against fat. The formula is in fact extremely effective for people who suffer from cold, slow metabolism. It is much less effective for overweight people who have red faces and fiery constitutions, since the Ma Huang only serves to cause more heat. Therefore, the thermogenic principle works for many people, but not for all people, and the herb can be harmful if abused or used excessively.

Many people have been attracted to Ma Huang because of its stimulating effect. It contains substantial amounts of ephedrine and pseudoephedrine, both central nervous system stimulants. Being a CNS stimulant, Ma Huang stimulates the adrenals, lungs, mind, and general energy.

The dangers of relying on Ma Huang for energy, though, cannot be overemphasized. Ma Huang is a stimulant and must be used very cautiously. It does not provide any *qi* to the body. In fact, it diverts energy away from the internal organs. This diverted energy can burn calories, relieve the surface, and clear the sinuses, but in a weak individual (a person low in *qi*), this cannot be sustained for long without causing exhaustion and other adverse side effects. If it is necessary to take Ma Huang for any sustained period of time, it should be a requirement that tonics be provided as well. In particular, Ma Huang appears to deplete the Kidneys. Therefore, it is wise to provide

Kidney *yin* tonics such as Prepared Rehmannia, Lycium Fruit, Ligustrum, and Schizandra. Furthermore, Pueraria Root seems to modify many of the side effects of Ma Huang while enhancing its beneficial effects. Therefore, Pueraria Root is almost always used with Ma Huang in Asian herbalism.

Chrysanthemum (no stars). The flower of a special variety of Chrysanthemum is used in China to improve circulation in the head and face and is thus used for headaches and sinus conditions. Since it has a cooling action, it is used to relieve red, swollen eyes caused by smog and summer heat.

Fantastic Tonic Herbal Formulations

Only a few Chinese supertonic herbs are used singularly: Panax Ginseng, Ganoderma (Reishi), Dang Gui, Acanthopanax (Siberian Ginseng), Notoginseng, American Ginseng, Ginkgo, Gynostemma, and Astragalus. These herbs are considered to be so great, so balanced, and so safe that they can be used with great benefit, over a long period of time, without auxiliary herbs. A few others, such as Deer Antler, Polygonum, Royal Jelly, and Cordyceps, are also consumed solo, but less commonly.

By far the majority of Chinese herbs are combined into formulations. Chinese herbal formulations contain from two to fifty herbs. Many of the formulas in common use today are classical combinations that have been used for centuries. Many others have been developed in recent times based on current needs and current research and information.

Formulations are constructed on age-old principles. Generally, certain combinations of herbs have been found through the centuries to have actions that are greater than the actions of the individual herbs used alone. Basic building blocks of formulations are known as entities and generally consist of from two to five herbs. An entity will have a specific action in a formula. A formula will be a combination of from one to ten entities, although most formulations contain about five.

In addition, formulations are usually constructed on the basis of "four positions." The four positions are known as the emperor, the minister, the assistant, and the servant. The herb or entity that plays the leading role in the formula is called the emperor. The emperor defines the primary function of the formulation. Some formulas may contain two or more emperors, meaning that they contain two or more primary functions. The minister is the herb or entity that provides primary support for the emperor and expands upon the original function. There will be at least one minister herb for each emperor herb. The assistant herbs and entities address a number of side issues and eliminate undesirable side effects. The servant herbs harmonize the ingredients and improve the taste of the formula.

Generally, these two methods are combined so that "entities" fill the "four positions." The overall effect of a formulation will rarely be determined by just one of its components. The synergism of the herbs is the defining quality of a formulation.

The creation of a formula is both an art and a science. Herbal formulations must be built upon the principles described, according to time-tested experience of herb combining and of appropriate proportions and quantities. Many of the formulations have not changed in hundreds of years. These are the classics. Most of the more modern formulations are actually modifications or combinations of classic formulations.

All of the formulations described in this chapter have been carefully crafted and have been used thousands, and in many cases millions, of times. See chapter 9 and the appendix, as well as the previous chapters describing specific herbs, for information on how to buy, prepare, and use herbs and formulas.

A Note on the Use of Ginseng and Codonopsis

Ginseng is used as the emperor in most *qi* tonic formulations. However, if the energy of Ginseng is considered to be too warm or stimulating, Codonopsis is usually substituted. This is standard Chinese tonic herbal practice. There is no dropoff in effectiveness when this is done if the Codonopsis is of high quality. Most of the formulations described in this chapter are available with either Ginseng or Codonopsis. Recently, other Ginseng substitutes have been employed, most commonly other varieties of Ginseng such as American Ginseng and Acanthopanax (Siberian Ginseng). The primary purpose of all these substitutions is to best balance the formula for the consumer.

THE CLASSIC SUPERTONIC HERBAL FORMULATIONS

The supertonic classics have been described in classic literature and used innumerable times through the centuries. Many of them date back to the second century A.D. No "classic" supertonic is newer than five hundred years old. All of these formulas are standards in the Chinese herbal system.

Four Major Herbs Combination

Four Major Herbs Combination is a fundamental formula in the Chinese herbal system. This is the primary *qi* tonic formulation and herb grouping ("entity") of Chinese tonic herbalism. Four Major Herbs Combination forms the foundation of numerous other formulations, in which other herbs are added. It is used as a major *qi* tonic by anyone wishing to increase vitality. Four Major Herbs Combination can improve the circulation of energy and the digestibility of many other herbs and foods. All four herbs in this superb formula are major Spleen tonics. Combined, they increase *qi* and improve digestion; and this is the primary function of this formula. It may also be used by those who are experiencing weak digestion, poor appetite, anemia, loss of voice caused by weak *qi*, borborygmus (growling abdomen), chronic fatigue, and general weakness. Due to their strong Spleen tonic effects, these four herbs help the body build muscle.

Composition: Ginseng or Codonopsis, White Atractylodes, Poria, and Licorice

Four Things Combination

Four Things Combination, sometimes called Dang Gui Four Combination, is the supreme blood tonic formulation of Chinese tonic herbalism. It is also an important *yin jing* tonic. It has been used for centuries as a nutritious, moistening blood tonic, which yields incredible results in restoring deficient blood and *yin*. In addition, it is an important blood-vitalizing agent which improves blood circulation in congested areas and dispels stagnant blood. It forms the foundation of a great many other formulations in Chinese herbalism. Four Things Combination is a famous women's blood tonic. It is moisturizing and may be used regularly to restore the *yin* and blood, to slow down aging, and to retard wrinkling and drying of the skin.

Composition: Dang Gui, Prepared Rehmannia, Ligusticum, and White Peony Root

Ten Complete Supertonic Combination

This is the original Da Bu Wan, or "superpill." It combines Four Major Herbs and Four Things and adds two other supertonics to make "the complete tonifying formula." This formula is a major energy and blood enhancer. It may be used by men or women to overcome chronic ailments due to *qi* and blood deficiency. It is used for fatigue, anemia, loss of appetite, and dry skin. It is routinely used for debility after an illness, surgery, or childbirth. It can strengthen eyesight in those with weakened vision due to fatigue. Furthermore, the formula is a formidable immune system enhancer, the most widely used basic formula for strengthening the immunity and resistance of immune-suppressed individuals.

Composition: Ginseng or Codonopsis Root, White Atractylodes, Poria, Licorice Root, Dang Gui, White Peony Root, Prepared Rehmannia, Ligusticum, Astragalus Root, and Cinnamon Bark

Ginseng and Astragalus Combination

Ginseng and Astragalus Combination has classically been called the King of Combinations. It is a giant among tonic formulations and is the premier energy tonic of Chinese tonic herbalism. It is classically said to promote the production and circulation of *qi*, strengthen the digestive system and improve nutrient assimilation, fortify the immune system, improve posture and the position of the organs, and is an excellent blood tonic. It is used as a tonic by anyone wishing to tonify or maintain a high level of *qi*, especially by those who are recovering from a chronic or acute illness or surgery.

Ginseng and Astragalus Combination is used by those suffering from chronic fatigue, malaise, general weakness, reduced resistance to disease, anemia, loss of body weight, a tendency to lose blood (as in excessive menstrual bleeding), and easy bruising. It is also used for edema, excessive phlegm, diarrhea, and abdominal bloating. In addition, it is used to strengthen the internal organs when they have prolapsed, resulting in conditions such as hemorrhoids, fallen uterus, varicose veins, and hernia.

Ginseng and Astragalus Combination supports the energy of weak people, restores energy to people who have exhausted themselves, and helps to restore immune function in those who have debilitated their immune system and developed chronic illnesses. It is currently the formula of choice in Japan to protect and rebuild *qi* in people undergoing chemotherapy and/or radiation therapy.

Composition: Ginseng, Astragalus Root, White Atractylodes, Dang Gui, Bupleurum, Cimicifuga, Dried Ginger, Licorice Root, Jujube Date, and Aged Citrus Peel

Ginseng Nutritive Combination

Ginseng Nutritive Combination contains all Three Treasures, and it has a tonifying and balancing effect by nourishing *yin* and *yang jing,* building blood, strengthening the *qi*, and stabilizing the Spirit (*shen*).

Ginseng Nutritive Combination is a superb general tonic, tonifying all Three Treasures—*jing, qi*, and *shen*—and all five primary organ systems: Kidneys (Water), Liver (Wood), Heart (Fire), Spleen (Earth), and Lungs (Metal). Ginseng Nutritive Combination is perhaps the quintessential Chinese tonic formulation.

Composition: Ginseng or Codonopsis Root, White Atractylodes, Astragalus Root, Poria, Dang Gui, White Peony Root, Prepared Rehmannia, Polygala Root, Aged Citrus Peel, Licorice Root, Cinnamon Bark, and Schizandra

Formula for Restoring the Pulse

A very popular tonic preparation called Formula for Restoring the Pulse is known for quickly rebuilding energy in those that have experienced trauma or surgery and for those recovering from illness. It has regained much popularity in recent years because of a host of clinical studies proving its efficacy in a wide range of disorders, all involving weakness.

Composition: Panax Ginseng, Cordyceps or Codonopsis Root, Ophiopogon Root, and Schizandra

Ginseng and Zizyphus Combination

Ginseng and Zizyphus Combination has been used for many centuries to tonify Heart *yin* and stabilize *shen*. Heart yin deficiency is characterized by mental and emotional instability, insomnia (troubled sleep, difficulty staying asleep), absent-mindedness, heart palpitations, constipation, and sores on the tongue or inside the mouth. This formula should be used for extended periods of time when treating insomnia.

Ginseng and Zizyphus Combination nourishes *yin jing* and pacifies the Spirit (*shen*), strengthens the Heart, and builds blood. Thus it tonifies all Three Treasures. This formula is specifically suited to those who are experiencing *yin* deficiency, especially if accompanied by hot, inflammatory symptoms (called false fire) and lack of stability of *shen*.

Composition: Ginseng or Codonopsis Root, Zizyphus Seed, Polygala Root, Biota, Poria, Asparagus Root, Ophiopogon Root, Rehmannia (raw), Dang Gui, Salvia, Scrophularia, Platycodon, Coptis, and Schizandra

Ginseng and Longan Combination

Ginseng and Longan Combination is the premier Spleen-Heart tonic of classical Chinese tonic herbalism. This formula tonifies two of the Three Treasures: it strengthens the *qi* (both the *qi* and the blood components) and calms the *shen*, allowing it to grow. This great *qi* and *shen* tonic formula has been used for centuries to increase vital energy and calm anxiety. It may be used to strengthen *qi* and blood that have become deficient due to major illness, chronic or acute bleeding, and/or mental or physical stress.

Some common symptoms for which this formula may be especially useful are anemia, insomnia (especially difficulty *falling* asleep), night sweats, prolonged menstrual bleeding, absentmindedness, confused thinking, palpitations, impotence, irregular menstruation, decreased vitality, and chronic fatigue. Ginseng and Longan Combination may be used for pallor, memory loss, and chronic conditions that reappear with an absence of inflammation. It is often used in programs that treat irregular menstruation, excessive menstruation, or continuous menstruation due to Spleen *qi* deficiency.

Composition: Ginseng or Codonopsis Root, White Atractylodes, Poria, Astragalus Root, Jujube Date, Licorice Root, Longan, Dang Gui, Zizyphus Seed, Polygala Root, Saussurea, and Dried Ginger

Lycium Formula

Lycium Formula is one of the greatest of all tonic formulations and is in particular a superb Primal Essence (*jing*) tonic. Lycium Formula influences primarily the Kidney functions (both *yin* and *yang*). It is also considered to be a Heart, Liver, and Spleen tonic. And Lycium Formula is an excellent blood tonic. It is used to strengthen the entire body, and as a brain tonic. It is highly regarded as a long-term sexual tonic for both men and women. Lycium Formula is said to strengthen the legs and the back. It is one of the few powerful vegetarian *yang jing* tonics in the supertonic class of Chinese herbalism and forms the foundation of a number of other major *jing* formulations.

Lycium Formula is literally called Return to Youth Formula. It is a famed rejuvenation formula. Other conditions that Lycium Formula is used to help balance are weakening and degeneration of the sense organs (especially eyesight and hearing), loss of memory and the ability to concentrate, general weakness, chronic fatigue, night sweats, impotence and general lack of libido, infertility, premature aging, and rapid degeneration. This superb Essence tonic is suited to men and women of all ages.

Composition: Lycium Fruit, Prepared Rehmannia, Jujube Date, Dioscorea Root, Poria, Broussonetia, Cistanches, Eucommia Bark, Morinda Root, Achyranthes Root, Fennel, Acorus, Polygala Root, Schizandra, and Cornus

Rehmannia Eight Combination

Rehmannia Eight Combination is one of the most important and commonly used *jing* tonics. It builds both *yin* and *yang jing*. This great tonic formula is particularly useful for *jing* deficiency in the middle-aged and elderly and is a superb tonic for maintenance of *jing* in older men and women. Rehmannia Eight has a broad range of applications.

It is a proven formula for the rehabilitation and strengthening of older people. It is famous for regulating blood sugar levels and has a long history of use for the control of diabetes and hypoglycemia. Rehmannia Eight is useful in the long-term treatment of sensory loss, fatigue, urinary incontinence, chills, lower back pain, premature ejaculation, impotence, absent-mindedness, memory loss, and chronic kidney and urinary disorders. It is used in Asia to regulate blood pressure. It is widely used for prostate problems in middle-aged and older men. A special note: Individuals with weak digestive function, especially those prone to loose stool, should take a Spleen *qi* tonic (such as Four Major Herbs Combination) to help with the digestion of Rehmannia Eight.

Composition: Prepared Rehmannia, Dioscorea Root, Moutan, Poria, Alisma, Cornus, Cinnamon Bark, and Prepared Aconite

Rehmannia Six Combination

Rehmannia Six Combination was created by removing the two *yang* herbs from Rehmannia Eight Combination. It is used as a *yin* tonic, especially to nourish the Kidney and to tonify its many classical functions. It is often used as an adjunctive formula for people who want to take a more *yang* tonic and who need to protect against overheating from the *yang* formula.

Composition: Prepared Rehmannia, Cornus, Alisma, Dioscorea Root, Moutan, and Poria

Lycium, Chrysanthemum, and Rehmannia Combination

This formula is used to improve vision that has degenerated due to deficiency of the Kidney and Liver functions. The formula is essentially the same as Rehmannia Six Combination, except that Lycium Fruit and Chrysanthemum flower have been added. The formula nourishes blood and *yin*, supplements the Kidneys, and benefits the Liver. It is used to relieve pain, swelling, and redness of the eyes and to relieve dizziness and blurring of vision due to eyestrain and fatigue. It can relieve tearing on contact with the wind and photosensitivity (intolerance to light) and other *yin* deficiency conditions treated by Rehmannia Six. While specifically benefiting vision, this is an excellent overall *yin jing* tonic.

Composition: Prepared Rehmannia, Dioscorea Root, Cornus, Poria, Moutan, Alisma, Lycium Fruit, and Chrysanthemum

Rehmannia and Schizandra Formula

Rehmannia and Schizandra Combination is another example of how a simple modification to a standard formula can change its function. This formula is created by adding Schizandra to Rehmannia Six Combination. It strengthens the Kidney functions in the same manner as does Rehmannia Six Combination, but in addition it strengthens the Lungs. It is believed that this formula improves the inspiration of *qi* by strengthening inhalation and the ability of the Lungs to "grasp *qi*." This formula is very effective for relieving severe coughing, but it need not be used solely for coughing. It is an excellent *jing* tonic.

Composition: Prepared Rehmannia, Cornus, Dioscorea Root, Poria, Alisma, Moutan, and Schizandra

Super *Yin*-Nourishing Formula

This formulation is designed to nourish *yin*, eliminate fire, and nourish the Kidney's *yin jing*. It is known in China as Da Bu Yin Wan. It is used as a tonic by those who have experienced extreme *yin jing* depletion and are manifesting inflammatory symptoms, a short temper, dryness, and night sweating.

Composition: Dendrobium, Plastrum Testudinus, Rehmannia (raw), White Peony Root, Anemarrhena, and Phellodendron Bark

Dang Gui and Astragalus Combination

Though this ancient formulation is extremely simple, being composed of just two herbs, it is considered to be one of the most effective tonic formulations ever created in China. It tonifies both blood and *qi*. When Dang Gui is added to Astragalus, Astragalus becomes much more of a blood tonic than when combined only with *qi* tonics. Together, these herbs are a powerful blood tonic that improves circulation and warms the extremities in people with cold hands and feet. This formula is used to treat fever due to weakness. It can be used to strengthen those who have become exhausted from lack of nutrition or from overwork.

Composition: Astragalus Root and Dang Gui

Dang Gui and Peony Formula

This formula is used as a blood tonic and "water-moving" tonic. Its most important functions are to nourish the blood, reduce bloating, strengthen digestion, strengthen the urinary function of the Kidneys, improve energy, and strengthen the back. It is often used for menstrual irregularity, difficult menstruation, and leukorrhea, all of which result from blood deficiency and poor fluid movement. It can also be used as a postpartum tonic to build energy and blood.

Composition: Dang Gui, White Peony Root, Ligusticum, White Atractylodes, Alisma, and Poria

Dang Gui and Gelatin Combination

This formula is a very powerful blood tonic aimed primarily at women. It is called a hemostatic. It prevents bleeding and breaks up blockages of blood, especially in the pelvic cavity. The formula can be used by women who are chronically or acutely anemic and those who are prone to miscarriage and habitual abortion.

Composition: Dang Gui, Rehmannia (raw), Ligusticum, White Peony Root, Donkey Skin Glue, Artemisia, and Licorice Root

Poria Five Combination

This famous classical formula is used to improve the utilization and circulation of fluids in the body. It promotes urination and is often used as a tonic to improve digestion and relieve fluid stagnation. It also has immune-potentiating activity and is especially beneficial to the digestive and urinary functions.

Composition: Alisma, Polyporus, Poria, White Atractylodes, and Cinnamon Twig

BUPLEURUM-BASED FORMULAS USED IN TONIC HERBALISM

Formulas based on the herb Bupleurum are among the most commonly used herbs in Chinese herbalism. They regulate the energy and have anti-inflammatory actions. They are commonly used in the early stages of a tonic herbal program to help harmonize the body. Many of them have profound stabilizing effects on the emotions. Here are some of the most useful Bupleurum-based formulas.

Minor Bupleurum Combination

Minor Bupleurum Combination is the most widely used classic herbal formula in Japan. It is one of the premier immune system tonics and is an extremely important formulation in Chinese herbalism. This formula is especially known for its benefits as a tonic for those who are recovering from colds and flu, and it is used throughout Asia as a preventive for these common ailments. It is used as an immunostimulant.

Composition: Bupleurum, Scutellaria, Pinellia, Ginger (fresh), Ginseng, Jujube Date, and Licorice Root

Bupleurum and Dragon Bone Combination

Bupleurum and Dragon Bone Combination is one of the primary antistress formulations used in Chinese herbalism. It is a superb mood stabilizer. It is primarily listed as a *shen* stabilizer and as a Liver tonic. It is known for its ability to help stabilize addictive-compulsive behavior and is widely used in the withdrawal from the addiction to smoking, drinking, and a large variety of addictive drugs by both lessening the cravings for the drug and reducing the common withdrawal symptoms. As an anticompulsive agent, this formulation can be used to control one's weight by helping to regulate the appetite. It is said to improve willpower, strengthen the mind, and reduce anxiety, frustration, and anger. It is widely used in Japan for chronic heart palpitations. It has a long tradition as a tonic to aid meditation. Those who are prone to loose stool will do better to use a version of the formula in which Rhubarb has been removed, since this herb has a laxative action.

Composition: Bupleurum, Scutellaria, Dragon Bone, Oyster Shell, Pinellia, Ginger (fresh), Ginseng, Poria, Jujube Date, Rhubarb, and Licorice Root

Bupleurum Formula

Bupleurum Formula is an excellent and reliable *shen*-stabilizing formulation. It is widely used to relieve tension, especially when it manifests as irritability and anger. In addition, this formula strengthens the constitution. It is therefore a superb formula for a wide range of the population, including all those who are overworked and/or overstressed.

Composition: Bupleurum, Uncaria, Dang Gui, White Atractylodes, Ligusticum, Poria, and Licorice Root

Bupleurum and Dang Gui Combination

Bupleurum and Dang Gui Combination, also known as Bupleurum Sedative Formula, is a *qi*, blood, and *shen* tonic; and it is a harmonization formula. Bupleurum and Dang Gui Combination nurtures, vitalizes, smooths, and regulates the flow of *qi* and blood. It normalizes digestive functions, and it is renowned for its ability to relieve a broad range of female imbalances.

Composition: Bupleurum, Dang Gui, White Peony Root, White Atractylodes, Poria, Ginger (fresh), Mentha, and Licorice Root

Bupleurum and Peony Combination

This formulation is used primarily by women to regulate their hormones and establish physiological balance. It has the additional function of establishing emotional balance, when hormone irregularities have caused an imbalance. It is used to treat irregular menstruation and many other female problems. It is the primary formula used in Chinese herbalism to eliminate premenstrual syndrome in women.

Composition: Bupleurum, Dang Gui, White Peony Root, Moutan, Gardenia, Mentha, White Atractylodes, Poria, Dried Ginger, and Licorice Root

RON TEEGUARDEN TONIC FORMULATIONS

Over the past two decades, I have created several hundred formulations for commercial consumption, and thousands more for individual clients. Most of these formulations were of a tonic nature. The following are the cream of that crop. They are all based on classical formulations and have all been used by thousands of people and have proved to be powerful toni-fying formulations.

Super Adaptogen

This formula contains most of the super adaptogens. It is a full-spectrum adaptogenic formulation which nurtures all Three Treasures and provides an abundance of the world's most potent phytonutrients. If someone were to take just one formula, this could be the one.

Composition: Gynostemma, Ginseng, Acanthopanax, Ganoderma, Lycium Fruit, Jujube Date, Eucommia Bark, Polygonum, Prepared Rehmannia, Longan, Astragalus Root, Schizandra, Polygonatum, White Atractylodes, Ginkgo Leaf, and Licorice Root

Adaptogen Energizer

This formula is similar to Super Adaptogen but contains fewer herbs. However, it contains more of each of the premier super-adaptogenics. Adaptogen Energizer increases mental and physical vitality both quickly and cumulatively. It expands the power of the body to adapt to all the stresses of life and strengthens the immune system. It helps overcome chronic fatigue and increases mental and physical endurance. In addition, this formula lowers cholesterol and helps reduce fat. It is good for men and women, old and young, and is excellent for the recovery from illness, surgery, and childbirth. It is an extremely potent *qi* tonic and is thus a top-notch athletes' formula. It even has anti-inflammatory activity.

Composition: Ginseng, Gynostemma, Acanthopanax, Schizandra, Astragalus Root, Ganoderma, Lycium Fruit, and Licorice Root

Supreme Protector

Supreme Protector is the ultimate Chinese protective formulation. It is composed of the three kings of defense in Chinese herbalism: Ganoderma, Astragalus, and Cordyceps. All protect the body and the mind in various ways. All are potent immune modulators and have powerful antistress activity. They also have antioxidant action and are highly adaptogenic. In addition, this formula powerfully tonifies all Three Treasures. This is indeed the supreme protector.

Composition: Ganoderma, Astragalus Root, and Cordyceps

Supreme Creation

Supreme Creation is the ultimate Chinese Primal Essence (*jing*) formulation. It is an elixir of unsurpassed quality. Supreme Creation is based upon a nine-hundred-year-old formula used by Chinese emperors to provide creative and procreative power. It is regarded as an extremely potent and well-balanced *yang jing* tonic suitable for most men and many women. The formula has gained a reputation for strengthening mental and creative power. It is believed to provide a fabulous creative spark. It is also a superb sexual tonic, an excellent athletes' formula, and a potent immunity booster.

Composition: Deer Antler, Placenta, Red Ginseng, Lycium Fruit, Schizandra, Epimedium, Dang Gui, Eucommia Bark, Morinda Root, Cistanches, Prepared Rehmannia, Cornus, Fennel, Dioscorea Root, Poria, Broussonetia, Acorus, Polygala Root, and Achyranthes Root

Diamond Mind

Diamond Mind is designed to strengthen and empower the mind. Each of the herbs in this formula has been used for centuries to improve concentration, focus, memory, and mental energy. By adding Deer Antler and Ganoderma, you have Super Diamond Mind, the ultimate mental rejuvenator and energizer.

Composition: Schizandra, Ginkgo Leaf, Polygonatum Sibericum, and Acanthopanax (Deer Antler and Ganoderma optional)

Buddha's *Yang*

Buddha's *Yang* is a powerful vegetarian *yang jing* tonic formulation. It is extremely potent. It tonifies the skeleton, strengthens the lower back and joints, and is a powerful sexual tonic. The formula is also extremely well suited to athletes who are looking for a potent *yang* tonic to increase strength, power, and endurance.

Combination: Epimedium, Cinnamon Bark, Prepared Aconite, Morinda Root, Eucommia Bark, Astragalus Root, Schizandra, Lycium Fruit, Cistanches, Cynomorium, Cnidium Seed, and Cornus

The Emperor's *Jing*

The Emperor's *Jing* is a famous and very special formulation which was used by an infamous Chinese emperor for *yang* primal energy. The Emperor's *Jing* is the most powerful *yang* tonic formulation money can buy. *Yang* tonics of this nature would traditionally be used by athletes to enhance physical power and performance and by those who wish to increase sexual vitality. These days, it is primarily used as a strengthening *yang* tonic beneficial to the whole system.

Composition: Deer Antler, Ginseng, Sea Horse, Sea Dragon, Epimedium, Cinnamon Bark, Prepared Aconite, Morinda Root, Eucommia Bark, Astragalus Root, Schizandra, Lycium Fruit, Polygala Root, Cistanches, Cynomorium, Cnidium Seed, and Cornus

Vital *Jing* Formula

Vital *Jing* Formula is a simple but very potent formula. It is used to strengthen the mind and body and to enhance the senses of vision and hearing. It is an excellent balance of *yin* and *yang* forces and will build genuine sexual vitality that will not be diminished.

Composition: Ginseng, Deer Antler, Schizandra, Lycium Fruit, and Licorice Root

Ron's Endocrine Tonic

This formula is designed to strengthen and regulate the endocrine functions. It contains herbs known to benefit the endocrine system. Ginseng has been well established as a pituitary-strengthening herb and is thus the primary herb of the formula (the pituitary is the master endocrine gland). Ginseng also benefits the functions of the Spleen. Most of the other herbs benefit the functions of the adrenal cortex and the gonads in terms of tonifying and regulating functions. This formula tonifies and regulates the entire endocrine system.

Composition: Ginseng, Prepared Rehmannia, Schizandra, Eucommia Bark, Dang Gui, Cornus, Dioscorea Root, Lycium Fruit, Poria, Licorice Root, Epimedium, and Jujube Date

Essence Restorative

Essence Restorative is a powerful Primal Essence formulation. It is suitable for those who require maximum restoration of Essence after extreme or prolonged stress, illness, or old age. It is particularly suitable for women who have been pregnant and who have just given birth. Essence Restorative tonifies Kidney Essence (*yin* and *yang*), builds blood, tonifies *qi*, and purges false fire. The formula is significantly strengthened by adding Placenta, which is the most potent *jing* restorative known to Chinese tonic herbalism.

Composition: Plastrum Testudinus, Eucommia Bark, Ginseng, Astragalus Root, Asparagus Root, Ophiopogon Root, Rehmannia (raw and prepared), Achyranthes Root, Phellodendron Bark, and Cornus (Placenta optional)

Frame Builder

Frame Builder can strengthen the structural framework of the body. The formula may be used by those who wish to strengthen bones, tendons, and ligaments. It is suitable for those who suffer chronic joint pain, lower back pain, knee pain, and so on. It is especially suited to those who are recovering from traumatic injury to bone, ligament, and/or tendon.

It can strengthen the lower back and knees and is an ideal tonic for those who experience lower back or knee pain due to exhaustion.

Composition: Eucommia Bark, Dipsacus, Drynaria, Morinda Root, Cistanches, Lycium Fruit, Poria, Dioscorea Root, White Atractylodes, Stephania, Angelica Anomala, Liquidamber, Notoptergium, Licorice Root, Clematis, Achyranthes Root, and Chaenomeles

Gecko Rockclimber

Gecko Rockclimber is designed to provide herbal nutrients for athletes and other highly active individuals such as dancers, actors, performers, and lovers. It may be used by those wishing to increase athletic and/or sexual power and by those interested in becoming generally more vital. It is suitable for those who have experienced adrenal exhaustion from chronic or acute stress, overwork, or sexual excess or by those whose work requires extraordinary physical prowess. It is designed for those wishing to strengthen the skeletal and muscular systems or for those experiencing weakening and/or withering of muscle and skeletal tissue. Gecko Rockclimber is a maximum potency formulation perfectly suited to those wishing to increase muscle mass without resorting to drugs or anabolic steroids.

Composition: Gecko, Panax Ginseng, Astragalus Root, Deer Antler, Morinda Root, Eucommia Bark, Lycium Fruit, Polygonum, Dang Gui, Dioscorea Root, Ligustrum, Donkey Skin Glue, Dipsacus, White Peony Root, Cornus, and Glycyrrhiza

Lucky Lixir

This is an excellent traditional *qi* tonic. It is used to promote growth, build resistance, and stabilize anxiety.

Composition: Royal Jelly, Astragalus Root, Cinnamon Twig, Jujube Date, White Peony Root, Dried Ginger, Licorice Root, and Maltose

Magu's Secret

Magu's Secret is a combination of wonderful tonic herbs traditionally used by the beautiful women of the Orient. It is said that the goddess of beauty and eternal youth, known as Magu, drank a tea of these great herbs every day to maintain her beauty, and offered them to the women of the world to benefit them in health and beauty.

Magu's Secret contains eight of the herbs associated with beauty in the Orient. A blood tonic, it is a blood-cleansing and blood-harmonizing formula and is said to contain all Three Treasures. It is a mildly *yin* formula especially suitable for women and men who wish to build blood, purify and enrich the skin, and enhance beauty from within.

Composition: Dang Gui, White Peony Root, Schizandra, Longan, Lycium Fruit, Cinnamon Twig, Albizzia Bark, and Coix

Magu's Treasure

In China, Magu is revered because of her warmth and deep beauty and also because she remained eternally young. Magu's Treasure is a combination of nothing less than the very finest tonic herbs available in the world, specifically designed as the ultimate women's tonic. It is composed of virtually every superior herb traditionally used by the most beautiful and wealthy women of the Orient.

Magu's Treasure is fundamentally a deep Essence tonic with strong blood tonic qualities. It contains all Three Treasures— *jing, qi,* and *shen*. It is believed in the Orient to be beneficial to all the functions of a woman. Magu's Treasure is the perfect balance of *yin* and *yang*, suitable for virtually all healthy women who wish to remain young and beautiful.

Composition: Deer Antler (tips), Placenta, Pearl, Royal Jelly, Dang Gui, White Peony Root, Schizandra, Lycium Fruit, Longan, Codonopsis Root, and Cynomorium

Yanlin's Beauty Formula #1

This formula was developed by my wife, Yanlin, who based it on a formulation described in a Chinese imperial book on beauty. It contains all the major beauty herbs used by Chinese royalty to promote beautiful skin and prevent aging.

Composition: Pearl (powder), Codonopsis Root, Schizandra, Dang Gui, Dendrobium, Lycium Fruit, White Peony Root, Peach Kernel, Asparagus Root, Sesame Seed, and Longan

Schizandra Lady's Sexual Elixir

This formula will awaken dormant energy and increase sexual sensitivity. It will enhance the development of orgasm and intensify the experience. It will also help produce sexual fluids. This is an excellent sexual tonic for women. It is warm but not overly so. Women who want even more sexual power may try adding half an ounce of Epimedium.

Composition: Schizandra, Longan Fruit, Deer Antler, Lycium Fruit, Morinda Root, Polygala Root, Dioscorea Root, Dang Gui, and White Peony Root

Peaceful Spirit Formula

Peaceful Spirit Formula is a supreme *shen* tonic, calming, soothing, and uplifting to the Spirit. The formula utilizes the Red Reishi mushroom (the Herb of Good Fortune) plus the greatest *shen* tonic herbs used by sages and wise people throughout the ages. Such a formula is considered in China to be able to help a person develop a peaceful, universal attitude and to strengthen the power of the mind. *Shen* Reishi is considered to be an excellent *shen* tonic for those who have suffered heartbreak, anxiety, excessive worry, or chronic fear and for those who have exhausted themselves emotionally and/or mentally. This is a pure *shen* tonic.

Composition: Ganoderma, Albizzia Bark, Spirit Poria, Bupleurum, White Peony Root, Jujube Date, Triticum, Polygonum, Longan, Acorus, Lycium Fruit, Schizandra, Salvia, and Licorice Root

Manifest *Shen* Formula

Manifest *Shen* Formula is designed to nurture *shen*. It is a Heart tonic. Manifest *Shen* Formula is the type of spiritual tonic used by the Daoist masters throughout Asia. It lifts the Spirit while steadying the emotions. It also nourishes the Lung and Kidney functions.

Composition: Ginseng, Ganoderma, Spirit Poria, Asparagus Root, Ophiopogon Root, Prepared Rehmannia, and Polygala Root

Profound Essence

Profound Essence is a very broad-spectrum formulation, with herbs that tonify all Three Treasures. Profound Essence is primarily a deeply restorative Essence tonic, focusing heavily on *yin* and *yang jing*. The overall effect of this formula is to replenish *jing* while preventing further loss of this primary Treasure. It is suitable as a long-term restorative *jing* tonic for those who have been exhausted by overwork, excessive stress, pregnancy, substance abuse, chronic pain, or chronic illness. It is also suitable for those who have reached midlife and who wish to replenish *jing* and prevent further degeneration.

Composition: Plastrum Testudinus, Rehmannia (raw), White Atractylodes, Poria, Dang Gui, Cuscuta Seed, Dipsacus, Eucommia Bark, Achyranthes Root, White Peony Root, Aged Citrus Peel, Phellodendron Bark, Anemarhena, Licorice Root, and Dragon Bone

Shou Wu Formulation

Shou Wu Formulation is a *jing* tonic designed to nourish the Kidney *yin* and to enrich the blood. The formula is headed by Polygonum. This product has the effect of improving adaptability, enhancing sexual and mental energy, strengthening the back and knees, nourishing hair growth, fortifying the senses, building blood, and producing sperm in men and increasing fertility in women. Shou Wu Formulation can be used as a basic Essence tonic by anyone, young or old, male or female. It is a superb antiaging and rejuvenation formula.

Composition: Polygonum, Dang Gui, Acanthopanax, Prepared Rehmannia, Aged Citrus Peel, Jujube Date, and Licorice Root

Dendrobium Primal *Yin* Replenisher

Dendrobium Primal *Yin* Replenisher is an extremely powerful *yin jing* tonic. It is for people who have severely depleted their *yin* reserves and are in serious health condition. *Yin* deficiency will lead to rapid aging, rapid deterioration of one's health, and premature death.

Composition: Dendrobium, Rehmannia (raw), Tortoise Shell, White Peony Root, Anemarrhena Root, Phellodendron Bark

Strength Builder

Strength Builder is designed to build and preserve Kidney *yin* and *yang*. It is a potent formulation designed to provide herbal nutrients for athletes and other highly active individuals. This formula may be used by those wishing to increase athletic and/or sexual power and by those interested in becoming generally more vital. It is suitable for those who have experienced chronic or acute stress, overwork, or sexual excess and for those who wish to maintain an active lifestyle. Strength Builder can be used to strengthen the skeletal and muscular systems and is particularly useful for those who use both their brains and their brawn to succeed.

Composition: Morinda Root, Polygonum, Eucommia Bark, Astragalus Root, Lycium Fruit, Dang Gui, Achyranthes Root,

Dioscorea Root, Ligustrum, Donkey Skin Glue, Dipsacus, White Peony Root, Cornus, and Licorice Root

Vitality Formulation

This formula is designed to quickly increase vitality. It is simple, but contains four of the greatest energy tonics. It is designed to increase both physical and mental energy as well as endurance. It is extremely effective.

Composition: Acanthopanax, White Atractylodes, Ginseng, and Schizandra

Immunity Booster Formula

This formulation is designed to boost immunity and build strong resistance. It may be used in conjunction with Supreme Protector. It contains seven of the most potent immune-enhancing herbs in the Chinese tonic herbal repertoire. It is suitable for anyone experiencing depressed immune responses.

Composition: Ganoderma, Shitake Mushroom, Astragalus Root, Poria, Codonopsis Root, Morus Alba Fruit, Ligustrum, and Licorice Root

Willpower

Willpower is based on a wonderful tonic herb now called Polygala, traditionally known as the Will Strengthener. Polygala is combined with herbs that strengthen *qi* and *shen*, helping us to remain "centered" during stress and thus allowing us to persevere through difficulties. Willpower can be used by anyone wishing to build willpower in order to achieve new heights and to break old habits, no matter how deeply engrained.

Composition: Polygala Root, Dragon Bone, Acanthopanax, Ophiopogon Root, Asparagus Root, Schizandra, Spirit Poria, Astragalus Root, Codonopsis Root, White Peony Root, Aged Citrus Peel, and Licorice Root

Young at Heart

This formula is a modern Heart tonic formulation using classic tonic herbs. It has been used clinically in China to improve coronary blood flow.

Composition: Salvia, Ligusticum, Crataegus, Notoginseng (raw), Dang Gui, and Astragalus

Young Lungs

This formula is a nourishing, immunoprotective Lung tonic. All of the herbs help clear the lungs of phlegm, moisten the membranes, and improve respiratory efficiency. This is an excellent tonic for those living in poor-air-quality environments and for those who have experienced weak lungs.

Composition: American Ginseng Root, Tremella, Glehnia, Schizandra, Ophiopogon Root, Prince Ginseng, and Licorice Root

Hair and Nails Formulation

Hair and Nails Formulation is composed of herbs that have been used for a thousand years by Chinese royalty to promote the growth of beautiful, healthy, strong hair and nails. The herbs are nourishing to the blood and thus provide needed nutrients to the hair and nails. The herbs also improve blood circulation, particularly the microcirculation. The formula removes toxins and stagnation and helps regulate hormonal functions.

Composition: Polygonum, Salvia, Rehmannia (raw and prepared), Dang Gui, Schizandra, White Peony Root, Chaenomeles, and Notoptergium

Hair Rejuvenation Formula

This is a well-known formula that is very effective. Like Hair and Nails Formulation, it features Polygonum. Its primary minister herb is Salvia, which improves circulation in the scalp. Hair Rejuvenation Formula contains Gastrodia as a major ingredient, which addresses "wind" conditions in the head, relieving tension in the scalp and improving smooth flow of blood and energy to the hair.

Composition: Polygonum, Gastrodia, Schizandra, and Ligustrum

Guan Yin's Precious Pill

This formulation is tonic to the female reproductive system. It is designed to stimulate female hormonal functions in such a way as to increase interest in sex and to promote fertility. It is rich in *yin* and *yang jing* herbs, antiaging herbs, and the primary fertility herbs of Chinese tonic herbalism.

Composition: Epimedium, Lycium Fruit, Schizandra, Eucommia Bark, Dang Gui, Prepared Rehmannia, Achyranthes Root, White Peony Root, Cuscuta Seed, Plantago Seed, Cynomorium, and Ligusticum

Easy *Qi*

Easy *Qi* is a relaxing yet energizing blend of ten superior herbs designed to relax, and thus enhance the free flow of energy, especially through the muscles of the back, shoulders, and neck. The formula is famous for its antistress action.

Composition: Bupleurum, Pueraria Root, Cinnamon Twig, Jujube Date, Licorice Root, Dried Ginger, White Peony Root, Angelica Tuhuo, Scutellaria, and Pinellia

Complete Immune Tonifying Formula

Complete Immune Tonifying Formula may be used by those with significant, chronic immune deficiency syndromes, and especially by those who exhibit signs of chronic deficiency fire. It is designed to be the primary immune-building and antimicrobial herbal supplement in an immunosuppressed individual's natural health program. It is a blend of the most powerful immune-modulating supertonic herbs, *jing* restorative herbs, and infection-fighting herbs. It is not a substitute for Western pharmaceutical drugs.

Composition: Ganoderma, Astragalus Root, Siberian Ginseng, Codonopsis Root, Plastrum Testudinus, Asparagus Root, White Peony Root, Isatis (root and twig), Morus, Platycodon, Lycium Fruit, Gentiana, Poria, Bupleurum, Asteris, Anemarrhena, Pinellia, Rehmannia (raw), Hypericum, Scute, Lonicera, Dried Ginger, Cinnamon Bark, and Licorice Root

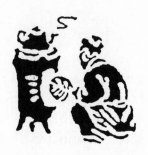

CHAPTER 8

Tonic Herbal Programs

The purpose of this book is to explain how to start and maintain an appropriate Chinese tonic herbal program that will be of true benefit with visible results. In developing a powerful and effective tonic program, you must consider several factors. First, your goals must be considered, since every person has different goals in life. A program will usually consist of a number of herbal preparations selected to help achieve certain long-range and short-range goals. You must also consider your own constitution, be it *yin* or *yang,* and of course you must frankly analyze your current condition and situation or have an expert analyze your condition for you.

The next thing to consider is the Three Treasures: *jing, qi,* and *shen.* According to your perceived strengths and weaknesses, and based upon your goals, you should select a *jing* tonic, a *qi* tonic, and a *shen* tonic, appropriately balanced according to the principle of *yin* and *yang.* Men and women generally take many of the same herbs because they are beneficial to everyone. Yet men and women are innately different biologically, physiologically, and even psychologically, and require certain specific herbs that help them develop optimal health and happiness.

By studying the first four chapters of this book, you should be able to determine how your Three Treasures are doing. In an ideal program, a person consumes herbs that help develop each of the Treasures optimally. A tonic herbal program does not focus attention solely, or even primarily, on symptoms. It focuses on the rebuilding of the energies that are the root of our existence. Therefore, *jing* is fundamental. Everyone should take a powerful *jing* tonic daily. There is no adult who cannot benefit from a *jing* tonic formula. As people grow older, they automatically become depleted of *jing*. Almost everyone needs *yin jing*, since this is the fuel of life. Many people also require *yang jing*. In fact, most people require both in some balance. Trying to determine the condition of one's *jing* and the proper balance of one's *jing* formula is central to the art of radiant health. *Jing* formulations are composed of the rejuvenation and antiaging herbs. A number of excellent *jing* tonic formulations were presented in chapter 7, each balanced slightly differently.

The *qi* tonic component is in many ways easier. The primary concern is whether you want more *qi* tonic herbs or blood tonics. Men generally use more *qi* tonics than women, and women use more blood tonics. The *qi* component includes most of the primary adaptogenic herbs that help us handle the stresses of life. The *shen* tonic component depends upon how much stress you are under and upon your spiritual aspirations. You may select formulations from those presented in chapter 7.

In addition, many people, when they first get into Chinese tonic herbalism, need to consume one Bupleurum-based formula. Bupleurum-based formulas are called *qi* regulators. They regulate the energy so that it does not "spike"; that is, the energy is controlled so that it does not fluctuate extremely. Many people experience wide fluctuations in their energy levels from minute to minute, hour to hour, day to day, or in some cases over the period of their monthly cycle. Any wild fluctuation is draining and needs to be stabilized. Many Bupleurum-based formulas are available, and a number of these have been described in chapter 7. Bupleurum-based formulas are used for the first year or so of a person's tonic program, after which the energy becomes self-regulating and the Bupleurum-based formulas become less necessary for most people or even unnecessary. In addition, one may wish to take one or more specific herbs or formulas to address certain specific problems. However, these should be selected with the help of an herbalist who understands remedial herbalism.

All this can be accomplished with one very sophisticated formulation prepared with excellent raw materials. The herbs are cooked as a soup and the resulting brew is consumed daily. This is an excellent approach and is most certainly the traditional one. Some people enjoy preparing tonic brews in this way, though it can be time-consuming and messy. Very few people these days prepare their own teas even once, much less consistently. However, there are now herbalists who prepare and prepackage herbal tonic teas for their clients. New technology allows these teas to be naturally preserved and easy to manage and consume. This supertonic tea generally forms the foundation of a program that may also include some of the fine prepared formulations described in chapter 7. This method has rapidly grown in popularity in the past few years.

The vast majority of people on tonic programs accomplish their goals by taking several commercially prepared formulations, combined in such a manner as to create a synergistic Three Treasures–based program. Virtually all of the formulations described in chapter 7 are available commercially in capsule or tincture form. This is, for most people, the easiest way to consume Chinese tonic herbs. Delivery systems will be described in more detail in the next chapter. The delivery system is the method of ingestion: in other words, liquid, capsules, and so forth.

GETTING STARTED WITH THE CHINESE TONIC HERBS

Getting started on a program of Chinese tonic herbs is easy. The two factors that make it easy are (1) the ready availability of excellent products in America at this time and (2) the safety of these products. The two primary concerns are (1) to select a delivery system that is comfortable for you and (2) to select a quality source. You will want to select a method that you can stick with for an extended period of time. You may have to experiment a bit on this, but once you find a delivery system that you can maintain, lock into that system.

Quality is of the utmost importance. Follow the guidelines presented throughout this book to find the best source of herbs you can find. The chemistry and energetics of different herbs can vary greatly, and many products on the market are not of high value. Your body, mind, and spirit deserve the best phytonutrients you can obtain. Higher-quality herbs contain more of the Three Treasures.

You want to focus on nurturing the Three Treasures, *jing, qi,* and *shen.* A good full-spectrum formula or a complete basic program provides a complete array of superior herbs consisting of a rich blend of the Treasures. These in turn will nourish all five elemental systems while balancing and regulating the *yin* and *yang* functions of the body and mind.

So where do you start? You cannot go wrong by taking any one of the following formulations. These formulations are suitable for just about anybody because they are considered to be neutral in terms of *yin-yang* balance. They provide an abundance of all Three Treasures.

- Ginseng Nutritive Combination
- Super Adaptogen

- Adaptogen Energizer
- Supreme Protector

If you choose to start off by taking one of the above formulations, you would need to consume an adequate amount of herbs to have a positive result within a reasonable period of time. Generally, if the herbs are concentrated spray-dried powders (as described in chapter 9), you would consume 1,000 to 4,000 mg (two to eight capsules), two or three times a day. These are not drugs and they are very safe. You may therefore feel free to experiment as to the amounts you consume and the frequency. Many people will find that smaller doses are most comfortable. Others will find that larger doses have a more profound impact more quickly. In general, you should start with a low serving in the beginning and build up. Most products provide suggested serving sizes and frequencies. Follow these instructions or the advice of a health practitioner.

Basic Herbal Programs

If you decide to become very serious about establishing radiant health by using tonic herbs, you will want to develop a full program. To do this, you will select several formulas, each with its own specific goal. The end result should be a well-balanced program that is rich in herbs that nourish the Three Treasures and the various organ systems of the body and is balanced to suit your constitution, from the perspective of *yin* and *yang*.

Here is a basic program that is suitable to just about anybody. These formulas are all considered to be neutral in terms of their *yin-yang* balance.

Jing—Shou Wu Formulation. Excellent alternatives: Essence Restorative, Ron's Endocrine Tonic, Rehmannia Six or Eight Combination, Lycium Formula.

Qi—Ten Complete Supertonic Combination. Excellent alternatives: Ginseng and Astragalus Combination, Ginseng Nutritive Combination, Ginseng and Longan Combination, Adaptogen Energizer, Super Adaptogen.

Shen—Peaceful Spirit Formula. Excellent alternatives: Manifest *Shen* Formula, Bupleurum Formula, Bupleurum and Dragon Bone Combination, pure Ganoderma.

Protection—Supreme Protector. Excellent alternatives: pure Ganoderma, pure Astragalus Root, pure Cordyceps.

Pick one formula from each category. These formulas provide the foundation of your Three Treasures program. Take two or three capsules of each, three times a day before meals. It's as simple as that!

The Traditional 100-Day "Cultivation" Period

In taking this program, you are establishing your personal Three Treasures program and have begun to build, or "cultivate," the Three Treasures in your body. Traditionally, it is believed that this initial stage of cultivation takes about one hundred days. However, you are likely to notice many positive changes in how you feel and look long before the first hundred-day period has run its course.

This "setup program" will accomplish all kinds of major tasks, including detoxification, purification of body tissues, balancing the major functions, building deep Essence (*yin jing*), establishing a fundamental level of protection, stabilizing the nervous system, and building *qi* so that you are revitalized and ready to progress further. This basic program is designed to regulate the *yin-yang* balance and to open communication in the five elements network.

This will all be initiated during the first hundred days. It is not necessary to concern yourself about developing a more sophisticated program at this stage. This program is already highly sophisticated. However, during the first hundred days, you should study up on the Three Treasures and on the principles of Superior Herbalism so that you will be ready to adjust your program for maximum benefit when you are ready to expand.

For the Adventurous and for Those in a Hurry

If right from the outset you have specific goals in mind, or just feel adventurous, you may wish to try one or more of the other superb formulations described in this book. You do this by adding other formulations to the foundation program. For example, women may wish to add additional Dang Gui–based formulas and men may add more *yang* tonic formulations. You may be interested in adding an energy-regulating formula from the Bupleurum group. In the following section, I will describe numerous programs that may serve as a guide for you. But always remember that all programs should be based on the Three Treasures if you wish to attain radiant health.

SPECIFIC PROGRAMS

In this section, I describe a number of basic programs. Based upon your condition and goals, you will be able to make decisions as to which herbs and formulas suit your needs. You can find more information on the formulas specified here in chapter 7 and more information on how to buy, prepare, and use herbs in chapter 9 and in the appendix.

Feel free to explore and combine these formulations in virtually any combination you feel is right for you so long as you remember to maintain balance in your program and to practice moderation. I believe it is always best to keep your program rather simple, but simplicity is a relative term determined by your level of expertise and discipline.

Adaptability Enhancement

We human beings are intimately interconnected with our environment. Any change in the environment influences us both physically and psychically. How we handle such changes, how we *adapt* to the changes in our environment and to the stresses of life, will be the determining factor in our health and well-being. Conversely, as we change, the environment around us will be influenced and will reflect our changes. The greatness of Oriental natural philosophy lies, to a great degree, in its subtlety and breadth of vision with regard to the connection between the human being and the environment. The tonic herbalist recognizes such environmental influences as the change of seasons, wind, heat, cold, dryness, moisture, and so on as fundamental causative factors in one's health as well as one's dis-ease.

Adaptability requires energy. The greater the stresses of life and the more dynamic the changes in one's life, the greater the requirement for adaptive energy. The very purpose of using Chinese tonic herbs is to aid the body-mind in its adaptive needs. The greatness of the Chinese tonic herbs lies in their *adaptogenic* quality; that is, their ability to enhance the body-mind's capacity to adapt optimally, accurately, and with endurance to changes in the environment, and thus to overcome the stresses of life.

By replenishing the energy of the cells, tissues, and systems that regulate our adaptability, we find ourselves capable of experiencing life at its fullest. We find ourselves with increased physical, mental, and emotional endurance. We find ourselves easily handling stresses that would exhaust others. We find ourselves to be resilient on every level. This adaptability allows us to lead a rich, broad, adventurous life.

When the body is working very well, it automatically adapts accurately. This is part of the miraculous self-regulatory mechanisms built into every cell of our bodies. This accurate adaptability is a key to radiant health. When you are radiantly healthy, nothing will bother you. If it's very hot, the body adjusts and you feel just fine. If it's cold, you adapt to that. People who adapt easily tend to be successful at life. But stress depletes this adaptive energy. Eventually, if you do not have enough adaptive *qi,* you start to maladjust, and sooner or later illness results. In addition, as we become less capable of adapting, we become more and more aware of the stress, and a vicious cycle occurs.

The Chinese tonic herbs are among the best tools on earth for combating stress. Obviously, it is better to avoid stress in the first place, or at least to submit ourselves to a minimum. Along with meditation, Yoga, and deep-breathing techniques, Chinese tonic herbs are the perfect natural way to help deal with stress. The herbs should not be taken like drugs to overcome stress. Tonics aren't meant to be used like that.

It takes energy to handle stressful events and forces. The tonic herbs provide that energy. If you are in a weakened condition and a stressful event occurs, of course you will feel more vulnerable and more stressed than if you had plenty of energy to deal with the problem. That is natural. By taking the adaptogenic herbs continuously, even when stressful factors are not strong, we can handle stress easily and overcome our problems with less agitation, even when circumstances become extremely stressful. The point, then, is to never run out of adaptive energy—to always have reserve energy so that when an emergency happens, you can deal with it without exhausting yourself.

ADAPTOGENIC FORMULATIONS

Most of the major *qi* tonic formulations are highly adaptogenic. Formulas such as **Ten Complete Supertonic Combination, Ginseng and Astragalus Combination**, and **Ginseng Nutritive Combination** are superb classic adaptogenic formulas. You may select the one that most appeals to you.

There are many modern formulations that feature one or more of the super Adaptogens. I have developed a number of such formulas. **Super Adaptogen** and **Adaptogen Energizer**, both described in chapter 7, are capable of building abundant adaptive *qi* and are the perfect herbal supplements for those who want to get the most out of life. They are pure adaptogenic formulations designed to provide an abundance of the kind of *qi* that allows us to perform optimally under all circumstances. Adaptogen Energizer and Super Adaptogen are safe for virtually anybody and can be consumed in large or small quantities.

Athletes' Programs

Ideally, everyone should exercise regularly in order to maintain good muscle tone and cardiovascular conditioning. A good exercise program can profoundly improve health. A person who takes exercise seriously is by definition an athlete. Athletes require special nutrition, and Chinese tonic herbs can play a very special role in an athlete's overall nutritional and conditioning program. Athletes all over the world have been using Chinese tonic herbs for many years, and in China itself tonic herbalism has played an important role in the training of martial arts practitioners for centuries.

In addition to working on the Three Treasures, which is the fundamental program for a long and healthy life, many individuals wish to add some special herbal products to their program. Any athlete can benefit from the supertonic herbs. An athletes' program will be oriented toward building a beautiful physique, maximizing performance, increasing strength and endurance, and helping attain deep health through exercise. The herbs are useful in helping to minimize damage, soreness, and injury and speed up recovery time.

You cannot maintain your youth, or attain radiant health, without engaging in healthy physical activity. It is essential that you maintain an exercise program for your entire life. Not only does exercise strengthen your muscles and skeleton, it benefits every system of the body, including the mind, when done properly. Balanced exercise will help you age much more slowly and suffer far fewer diseases and disorders. Americans are generally very aware of the need for exercise, and a good many have discovered how much better they feel and look by exercising regularly. There has been a health club explosion to meet this demand. In addition, running and bicycling are bigger than ever. Home exercise equipment now adorns many American homes and apartments. And people are finding all kinds of new and interesting ways to exercise and get in shape. Rock climbing, scuba diving, and mountain biking have all grown in popularity in the 1990s.

It is possible to get more out of your exercise by taking the Chinese tonic herbs. The herbs have a long history of being used by athletes. The art of athletic tonic herbalism is as fundamental and as old as the martial arts are in China—and that goes back over two thousand years. The tonic herbs were central to the Shaolin Temple training that was made famous in the television series *Kung Fu*. In real life, those Shaolin monks and trainees took (and still take) tonic formulas every day to build muscle, increase strength, sharpen concentration, build endurance, alleviate stress, relieve pain, and build willpower. These are all attributes that today's athlete needs as well. Whether you play basketball, tennis, golf, rugby, volleyball, or Ping-Pong, you can benefit from these herbs. If you go to the gym to get your exercise and do your aerobics, these herbs can help you get leaner and stronger faster. If you dance, the herbs can give you strength and endurance, reduce fat, and even help with your coordination.

I have known and worked with numerous athletes during my career as an herbalist. I have worked with professional football, basketball, and tennis players. I have put the world's greatest golfers on herbal programs. World-stature triathletes and cross-country bicycle racers use the tonics. Olympic and professional boxers use the tonics. Professional beach volleyball players use the tonics. Many of the world's most famous bodybuilders use them. The list goes on and on. I mention this just to let you know that you are not experimenting with something new and untried. All these athletes are very aware of the differences in how they feel and perform when they do something different. And the tonic herbs are something they really notice. There is absolutely no question that performances can be improved by the use of high-quality tonic herbs.

Athletes require different formulations based upon their physical constitution, current physical strengths and weaknesses, and the nature of their physical activities. Athletes often do well to see a professional and be put on a tonic program that optimizes the benefits. However, there are a number of great tonic formulas that can be used to improve athletic capability and skill. Here are some formulas beneficial to most athletes.

To Build Physical Strength, Power, and Endurance

Ginseng and Acanthopanax (Siberian Ginseng) are extremely popular among athletes around the world. Both build energy and endurance that athletes really notice. These may be used alone and there are many brands available. However, I advise all athletes to find the highest-quality Ginseng possible, since lower-quality products can be useless, and in some cases detrimental.

For even better results, athletes can now use more sophisticated formulas based on both long-standing knowledge and modern research. The adaptogenic formulas discussed in the previous section are perfect for athletes. They will provide an added dimension to an athlete's training and, ultimately, to the athlete's capabilities. Here are a few other formulas that can be of use to many athletes.

Gecko Rockclimber is a formula designed to build muscle and strength. If you take this formula while you are working out, your workouts will achieve more, and you will progress noticeably more quickly. In addition, it will strengthen both metabolism and respiration. It will build *qi,* blood, *yin,* and *yang.* In particular, your lungs will benefit from using this formula. The Gecko lizard has long been used by martial artists in Asia to improve the functioning of the lungs. It is said that Gecko increases the extraction of *qi* from the air we inhale, thus increasing lung power, energy, and endurance. This is a formula for the serious athlete.

Cordyceps may be used individually as an adjunct to Gecko Rockclimber. In China, Cordyceps is considered to be virtually essential for athletes who rely on strength, speed of foot, and endurance.

Strength Builder is very similar to Gecko Rockclimber. It, too, is a premium athletes' formula. Other formulas that athletes have used are **Lycium Formula, Supreme Creation,** and **Vitality Formulation**. All of these are excellent.

For Problems with the Bones, Tendons, Ligaments, and Joint Inflammation

Frame Builder is designed to help broken bones, torn ligaments, and torn tendons heal more quickly. It helps relieve inflammation in the joints and can therefore be used preventively by those who have soreness due to stress on the joints. It is especially good for helping relieve knee pain and for helping the knees to heal quickly and completely. It can be used all the time in moderate quantities. Or it can be used in large quantities during rehabilitation or when the problem is acute. See a doctor if you have pain, but these herbs will definitely help. There are other herbs that may be added to this formula to aid in the healing. Your herbalist will know what to add.

How to Use the Tonics to Build Athletic Prowess

Herbal supplements should be made from concentrated powders or liquids. Don't waste your time with raw powdered herbs that have not been concentrated—they are too weak. Take a little more than most people. I have found that athletes have big appetites not only for regular foods but for tonic herbs as well. That is natural, since the requirements of being an athlete are so high. You might start off a little slowly just to get a feel, but don't be afraid to take plenty. These herbs are safe, and they are extremely effective when you take enough. Their antioxidant and free-radical clearing capacity will be of tremendous benefit, and they will optimize tissue repair and growth.

Fertility

Fertility is generally associated with the *yin jing,* while potency is associated with *yang jing. Yin jing,* in this regard, represents the hormones and other substances and fluids related to reproductive functioning and fertility. *Yang jing* represents sexual drive and functioning. In reality, both aspects of the Kidneys must be functional if fertilization is to take place. Deficient circulation in the uterus, for example, is often believed to be the cause of female infertility. This condition is called a cold uterus by the Chinese, and this is treated by "warming the uterus," which is accomplished by increasing blood flow through the pelvic basin and the reproductive organs contained therein. Blood is *yin,* but the warmth and circulation are *yang.* Without both, fertilization and pregnancy cannot succeed.

Male Fertility

Male fertility is generally believed to be fostered by the use of *yin* and *yang jing* formulations, especially ones containing Polygonum, Deer Antler, Astragalus, and any number of the other male sexual tonics like Epimedium and Cistanches (see the section on male sexuality).

An excellent formula that men may use to increase sperm production and fertility is **Shou Wu Formulation,** which may be used with a separate supplement of Astragalus. Fifteen hundred milligrams of Shou Wu Formulation and five hundred milligrams of Astragalus, taken three times a day for several weeks are a typical dose.

Polygonum is used to increase sperm count and to tonify *jing.* Astragalus improves the *qi* of the sperm and has been shown to increase sperm motility.

If the man lacks sexual drive, a *yang jing* tonic would be advisable. A number of such formulations are described in the section on sexual tonics.

FEMALE FERTILITY

A woman hoping to increase her fertility should take a basic women's tonic formulation. These formulations will build blood and regulate the menstrual cycle. **Four Things Combination** or **Ten Complete Supertonic Combination** is perfect for building blood and strengthening a woman's constitution. They will help to regulate female hormonal functions and increase fertility.

In addition, a woman seeking to become pregnant may take **Guan Yin's Precious Pill** to increase fertilization potential. This sophisticated formulation increases both *yin* and *yang jing* in a woman. It improves blood and *qi* circulation to the pelvic organs, warms the uterus, and increases sexual drive. It thus promotes fertility. It prevents miscarriage during the first weeks of pregnancy.

There are many causes of infertility. It is wise to seek professional advice. Chinese tonic herbs can be very useful, and the high rate of success people achieve using these herbs is astounding.

Beautiful Hair

Beautiful hair is one of the most striking features a woman or man can possess. Healthy, beautiful hair, like the skin, requires internal nutrition in order to flourish. The Chinese have long known about certain herbs that nourish the hair. Polygonum is by far the most famous. It has been China's internal and external hair tonic for over fifteen hundred years! It is one of herbalism's premier blood tonics. It is also one of the major Kidney *jing* tonics. It is famous as a rejuvenating herb for the whole body and the hair in particular. It has moistening qualities that make the hair shine, and it is said that constant consumption of Polygonum will return the hair to its natural color and youthful luster.

However, Polygonum is not the only herb that improves the condition of the hair. When combined with certain other herbs, Polygonum's power to generate and nourish the hair is increased.

Hair and Nails Formulation, described in chapter 7, is specifically used to nurture beautiful hair. The herbs in this formula improve circulation to the scalp, nourish the hair follicles, and reduce inflammation. It has proved to be very effective at stimulating new hair growth. Many people have claimed that their hair started growing again after taking this formula for several weeks.

Another popular formula used by many beautiful women in China is **Hair Rejuvenation Formula**. This formula is used to prevent premature graying and premature loss of hair as well as to beautify the hair itself by providing it with special nutrients. It is especially good for those who feel they are losing hair due to stress.

Immune-Boosting Formulations

Chinese tonic herbs have profound immune-boosting characteristics. Frankly, any program of high-quality Chinese tonic herbs will help to build the immune system so that your resistance is improved. This is, of course, of fundamental interest to those who wish to build radiant health, which we defined as "health beyond danger." Those who desire to specifically address their immune capacity have a great many wonderful options among the Chinese tonic herbs. Here are a few suggestions to help you on your way.

Take Ganoderma and Astragalus every day as a routine part of your health program. I recommend this to every one of my personal clients. And I follow my own advice. I take both these herbs in significant quantities every day, and even more when I travel or am exposed to ill people and large crowds in closed areas (such as packed Asian subways, concert halls, and airplanes). These two supertonics are unmatched as immune potentiators. Be sure that what you are taking is high-quality. Reread the sections on these herbs in chapter 5 so that you understand what you are getting. I recommend at least 1,500 mg of each concentrated powder a day. I take 3,000 mg a day of each and double that when I need to. These are very safe herbs.

Consider adding other tonic herbs that have been shown to have powerful immune-potentiating activities. Cordyceps, Codonopsis, Gynostemma, and others have profound immune-modulating activity, which will help build the immune system. Remember, you do not want to wait to become ill and then have to take medicinal ("inferior") herbs like Goldenseal or Echinacea. This is too late. Each time you get sick, you are damaging your body and shortening your life (not to mention lost work and play days).

Ginseng and Astragalus Combination, Ten Complete Supertonic Combination, and **Ginseng Nutritive Combination** have all been discussed. These are major immune-strengthening formulas. Any one of these may be your first choice as a daily immune booster. They are unbeatable at building the immune system back to optimum strength. These formulas are suitable for all individuals who wish to build and maintain their resistance. They are also primary formulas for those suffering from chronic fatigue syndrome, HIV infection, and other immune deficiency conditions. They may be safely used along with drugs, under a doctor's supervision.

Another primary formulation you should consider is

Supreme Protector, which contains Ganoderma, Astragalus, and Cordyceps. This is Chinese tonic herbalism's supreme combination of immune-boosting supertonic herbs. This formulation is commercially available. It is extremely safe and effective.

Immunity Booster Formula, another commercially available formulation, is designed to boost immunity and build strong resistance. It may be used in conjunction with Supreme Protector. It contains eight of the most potent immune-enhancing herbs in the Chinese tonic herbal repertoire. It is suitable for anyone who is experiencing depressed immune responses or who may be exposed to infectious situations.

Minor Bupleurum Combination is frequently used to prevent relapses of colds and flus. It is used as an immunostimulant. It is used as a tonic and preventive by those with upper respiratory allergies and by those who are prone to sore throats. It is also considered to be a major Liver tonic. Minor Bupleurum Combination is one of the primary agents used in Japanese medicine for the treatment of chronic hepatitis. It has been found to be effective in the treatment of chronic fatigue syndrome. In these and other disorders, it has been shown to regulate the immune response in order to effect optimum healing. A slightly modified version is now widely used in HIV programs in Japan. It should be used along with major immune-building herbs like Ganoderma, Astragalus, and Cordyceps.

CHINESE TONIC HERBS AND HIV

Many herbal practitioners have been exploring the possibility that people infected with the human immunodeficiency virus (HIV) may benefit from the use of herbs and other safe, natural products. There is no known cure for this condition, and no Chinese tonic herbalist would claim otherwise at this time.

However, great progress has occurred in the past few years in the Western medical field. There are increasing reports of individuals who are becoming apparently virus-free. Chinese tonic herbs may still be included in an immunosuppressed individual's program because the tonic herbs are health-promoting. They're good for everyone, especially those who need an extra boost.

In the Orient, the Chinese tonic herbs and herbal formulations are believed to strengthen the body and mind, enhance immunity, improve functioning of the various organs, relieve stress, and generally improve well-being and even to lengthen life if consumed regularly over a long period of time. It is imperative that the immunocompromised individual realize that it is not enough to eliminate the virus and other microbes if health is to be restored. The *jing* must be protected and rebuilt, *qi* production must be encouraged, and all functions of the body must be fortified and harmonized, even if the virus is otherwise eradicated. Tonic herbalists in America use the Chinese tonic herbs to enhance normal functions. The herbs used are very safe, having been used for thousands of years, and their safety has been further verified by modern studies in Japan, China, and elsewhere.

It is highly encouraged that all people who are HIV positive visit their health practitioners regularly and inform them of all Chinese herbal products used. Do not consider the herbs to substitute in any way for treatment prescribed by the practitioner. For example, if you have been placed on AZT and/or other drugs, you should continue to follow the prescribed regimen under your health practitioner's supervision.

A Chinese tonic herbal program is an individual thing. It is based upon the traditional concept that a strong, adaptable system will prove in most cases to survive, even under adverse conditions. Therefore, a "general supertonic" formula is usually suggested. There are many such great general tonic preparations available today, and these can be used whether or not one is suffering from immune deficiency. **Ginseng and Astragalus Combination** is an example of such a supertonic formulation, and **Complete Immune Tonifying Formula** is a perfect example of a full-spectrum formula designed specifically for HIV-infected individuals. Thousands of HIV-positive individuals have used these products without negative side effects.

Complete Immune Tonifying Formula may be used by those with significant, chronic immune deficiency syndromes, and especially by those who exhibit signs of chronic deficiency fire. These fire symptoms include chronic fevers, hot flashes, chronic inflammatory conditions, redness and swelling of the throat and sinuses, and red blemishes. Other formulations may be useful or even required, as directed by an herbalist. This product is to be used with a health practitioner's consent when necessary, such as during acute stages of infection or when the practitioner determines that all consumable substances require his or her consent. All relevant studies conducted in China, Japan, the United States, and elsewhere indicate that Complete Immune Tonifying Formula may be used safely and effectively along with modern Western drugs, a practice that may yield the best results. Such combining of Western therapies with Chinese tonic herbs is known as Fu Zheng therapy, which has attained notable acceptance around the world.

This general tonic formulation is usually supplemented by a superbooster herb or formula. The **Supreme Protector** is precisely such a formulation.

Lower Back and Knee Problems

Lower back pain, or lumbago, is one of the most common ailments in our society. When the Kidney energy is depleted, a simple action may cause the back to go into spasm. A simple awkward movement is not the action that causes one's back to "go out," however. Most often, when a person's back goes into acute spasm, or the person displaces or ruptures a disk, that person has recently experienced severe stress. The stress exhausts the adrenals, and after the stress is over and the person is able to relax, the adrenals shut down for a period of time while the body rebuilds its hormonal supplies. During this time, the body is not able to handle additional severe stress, and a simple action can result in injury to the back. In the Orient, it is not considered sufficient to confine treatment to physical therapy on the back. It is also considered necessary to rebuild the Kidney energy so that the root of the back injury is eliminated and so that the back is strengthened from within. Backs heal only very slowly, if at all, if the Kidneys are not nurtured along with direct work on the injured tissue itself. Strengthening the back from within by tonifying the Kidney energy can result in complete recovery.

The knees and the ankles, too, are under direct influence of the Kidneys. These joints are most often injured when a person has been under chronic stress and then encounters a severe acute stress. These joints are, like the lower back, also weakened by excessive sexual activity, which depletes the Kidney energy. It is said that sexual activity is excessive if the knees become weak or the back aches after sex. Strengthening the Kidneys, of course, strengthens sexual energy and increases one's capacity and protects the lumbar area and the knees. The feet and ankles often hurt spontaneously when the kidney energy has been depleted.

Generally, any high-quality, properly balanced *jing* tonic will strengthen the back and knees. Most people require both *yin* and *yang*. **Lycium Formula** is a perfect example of such a formula. So are the restorative formulations **Essence Restorative** and **Profound Essence**.

Frame Builder is a formula that has been specifically designed to strengthen joints, especially the lower back, knees, and ankles. It is based on the herb Eucommia, which has been used for centuries by martial artists to strengthen and help heal joints. This is a remarkably effective formula for those who have suffered injury. It can significantly hasten recovery.

Men's Programs

In Chinese herbalism, it is said that men are ruled by *qi*, while women are ruled by blood. This means primarily that men need to take *qi* tonics and *yang* herbs, while a woman should take primarily blood tonics and *yin* herbs. Men require an abundance of *qi* and *yang*, but this does not mean that a man does not need blood and *yin*. In fact, the opposite is true. If a man is blood deficient, he will be weak and have low resistance to disease. If he lacks *yin*, his basic life force will be diminished. A man must be very careful not to abuse his *yin* energy by becoming too *yang* or by taking too many *yang* tonics.

However, men thrive when they have plenty of *yin* and *yang* energy. Therefore, men's tonic programs tend to focus first on building *yin* and *qi*, and once the *yin* is developed, the focus may be placed on building and maintaining strong *yang* reserves. In general, then, men who have full *yin* reserves may take large amounts of *yang* herbs. These are the power herbs and the sexually strengthening herbs.

Men stay young by staying in good athletic condition and good sexual condition. The sexual hormones nurture the cells of the body and prevent aging. It is not necessary for a man to have sex all the time, or even at all. But it is necessary to maintain the sexual organs in a healthy state, or aging will set in prematurely.

Excellent formulas for men include **Ginseng Nutritive Combination, Lycium Formula, Buddha's *Yang*, Shou Wu Formulation, Strength Builder, Rehmannia Eight Combination, Ron's Endocrine Tonic,** and **Supreme Creation.** Supreme Creation is the most potent for most men, but all are powerful. Of course, men need other factors in their life besides hormone-regulating formulas. For example, every man should consume **Supreme Protector** daily.

Mental Energy

In all of history, the human mind has never been more universally challenged. The requirements of living in the modern era include the exertion of an enormous amount of mental energy. Just dealing with our bills is more mind-boggling than any math I ever encountered in high school. And the day we finally figure out how to use a computer program, a new version is released, and we have to learn all over again. Everybody is working with computers and they require logic and focus. All the so-called conveniences of the modern era are designed to use the mind rather than the body. For exercise, we go to a gym where we pump a computerized unit instead of working in a field. We get more work done because of the computers, but that means we have to keep more on our virtual desktop than would have been conceivable a decade ago.

So in this explosive, breakthrough period of mind over matter, high-tech machine over body, it is imperative that everybody remain in top condition *mentally* at all times. As a result, there has been an explosion of interest in mind tonics in the past several years. The popularity of coffeehouses reflects our current need as a society to form more mental energy. But coffee may not be the best way to get the most out of our minds.

Many formulas contain mind-strengthening herbs, but formulas such as **Super Adaptogen** and **Adaptogen Energizer** are rich in these particular substances. A formula specifically designed as a mind tonic is **Diamond Mind**, which should have quick and profound results.

BRAIN RESTORATIVE FORMULAS

Sometimes the mind is too fatigued to be clear. Confusion is often the result. Confusion allows emotions to rule our lives rather than *shen*. In that case, there is a *shen* type of formula that is very effective at revitalizing the mind. This type of formula calms the mind and simultaneously improves circulation to the spinal cord and brain. In Chinese herbalism, the mind is said to be controlled by the Heart function. The Heart energy is what is being manipulated by these "peaceful spirit" formulas. The Kidneys are said to control the brain—its health and energy. Therefore, when the Kidneys are exhausted, the mind becomes weak. Exhaustion of the body will lead to exhaustion of the mind and vice versa. Anything that depletes the Kidneys will ultimately make the mind weak. The Kidneys are the power supply to the brain. Excess in sexual activity, stress, drug use, fear, and emotionalism can weaken the mind as a secondary effect because such excess depletes the Kidneys. Therefore, it will be necessary to tonify the Kidneys as well as the Heart. An appropriate *jing* formula in combination with **Peaceful Spirit Formula** will do the trick.

Peaceful Spirit Formula can strengthen the mind and increase wisdom. It has the Reishi mushroom (Ganoderma) as its lead herb and Polygonatum sibericum as the minister. Reishi strengthens the Heart and promotes wisdom. Polygonatum sibericum rejuvenates the mind.

Do not expect the peaceful spirit variety of healthy brain pills to be stimulating or to replace your cappuccino. These formulas are actually sedative. But after a month of taking them, your mind will be very strong. You will be able to think clearly and with tremendous endurance.

If you want stimulation, use the power herb formulations such as **Adaptogen Energizer, Super Adaptogen,** or **Supreme Creation.** These herbs will stimulate the mind quickly without exhausting it. They will replenish as you go. I recommend that you take these herbs in the morning and the Peaceful Spirit Formula at night. In this way, you will rejuvenate your mind, and within a short time you will feel sharper, more alert, and more focused. You might even be more intelligent.

Recovery from Illness, Accidents, and Surgery

There are a number of formulations used to aid in the recovery from illness, accident, or surgery. These formulations have been clinically used tens of thousands of times in China and Japan. Numerous studies have been conducted on the four formulations recommended below, and in each case the patients recovered more quickly and completely than patients who did not take such formulas.

Ten Complete Supertonic Combination has been used by millions of people who were in a recovery situation. The formulation is extremely effective at promoting healing, building blood, strengthening the immune system, increasing energy, strengthening the appetite, and improving microcirculation. It is favored when there has been blood loss.

Ginseng and Astragalus Combination is equally popular as a recovery formulation. It, too, promotes rapid healing and quickly increases energy. It is favored for recovery from illness that had depleted the body.

The Formula for Restoring the Pulse is extremely mild, yet extraordinarily effective. It is therefore suited to young and old alike. It contains premium herbs, but the formula may be adapted to the individual. Sometimes it includes Ginseng, sometimes Codonopsis, and sometimes Cordyceps. It always includes Ophiopogon and Schizandra. It is now the most widely used recovery formula in hospitals and at convalescent homes in China. It is favored when recovering from a depleting illness.

Ginseng Nutritive Combination is another extremely effective recuperative formula. It is especially effective in helping to strengthen a person after surgery or illness and for women after childbirth. It builds resistance to disease by tonifying the immune system.

In practice, all four formulas are commonly used in China during rehabilitation from serious illness, surgery, or traumatic injury.

Rejuvenation Formulations

Two classical formulations have been used for many centuries to rejuvenate the body and mind and to maintain youthful vigor. They are among the greatest tonic herbal formulations ever designed. I have found them to be almost unfailing in their effectiveness when taken consistently over a reasonable period of time.

Ginseng Nutritive Combination is arguably the greatest general Three Treasures tonic in Chinese classical herbalism. It has been my favorite for many years. It is a superb general tonic, tonifying all Three Treasures and all five primary organ systems. Virtually anybody can benefit from this formula.

Ginseng Nutritive Combination has been used for centuries as a tonic for poor memory, anxiety, insomnia, night sweats, absentmindedness, weakness from overexertion, fatigue, dry skin, palpitations, premature ejaculation, impotence, infertility, hair loss, and blood-deficient pallor. This is a great rejuvenation formula.

Lycium Formula is one of the greatest of all tonic formulations and is in particular a superb *yin* and *yang jing* tonic. This formula influences primarily the Kidney functions (both *yin* and *yang*). It is also considered to be a Heart, Liver, and Spleen tonic. In addition, Lycium Formula is an excellent blood tonic. Traditionally, Lycium Formula has been called Return to Youth

Formula, and for good reason. It is used to strengthen the entire body and is especially respected as a brain tonic. It is highly regarded as a long-term sexual tonic for both men and women. It is also used to strengthen the legs and the back and is a major rejuvenation formula.

Lycium Formula has traditionally been used to help correct the following conditions: weakening of the sense organs, loss of memory and the ability to concentrate, general weakness, chronic fatigue, night sweats, impotence and general lack of libido, infertility, premature aging, and rapid degeneration.

Lycium Formula forms the foundation of a number of other major *jing* formulations including Supreme Creation, which is the "imperial version." Supreme Creation adds Deer Antler, Placenta, and Ginseng to the mix. This superb tonic is suited to men and women of all ages.

Super Shou Wu Combination is a superb rejuvenation formulation. It is suitable to anybody who is experiencing chronic fatigue, depression, loss of sexual drive, or premature aging. It can form the base of a superb tonic program. This formula contains Siberian Ginseng, so it can have an immediate energizing effect on many people. It is extremely well suited for older people who want to regain their zest, but it is also great for young people who are exhausted.

Restorative Formulations

Restorative formulations play a critical role in the rejuvenation of those people who have already exhausted themselves and have seriously drained their deepest energy reserves of *yin* and *yang jing*. These formulas restore the deepest energies of the body. They generally aim deeper than rejuvenation formulas, which aim deep, but also aim to nourish all levels of energy. Those who have burned themselves out generally cannot recover with rest alone. They require a restorative formula. Taking these formulas is like recharging a drained or almost dead battery.

All of the following formulations are composed primarily of Kidney tonic herbs, sources of *yin jing*. This is because *yin* is the fuel of life, and it is the depletion of *yin* that results in chronic fatigue, or actually, chronic *exhaustion*. Some restorative formulations contain *yang jing* herbs as well. In addition, all the formulations contain at least one astringent herb used to "lock" the *jing* in the Kidneys. This is an essential component. It prevents the leaking of energy that causes chronic fatigue.

Restorative formulations may be consumed continuously until energy is fully restored. Older people can take restorative formulations on an ongoing basis.

Rehmannia Eight Combination is one of the most important and commonly used Essence (*jing*) tonics. It builds both *yin* and *yang jing*. This great tonic formula is particularly useful for *jing* deficiency in the middle-aged and elderly and is a superb tonic for maintenance of *jing* in older men and women. Rehmannia Eight Combination has a broad range of applications.

Rehmannia Eight Combination is a proven formula for the rehabilitation and strengthening of older people. This formula is famous for regulating blood sugar levels and is used for the control of diabetes and hypoglycemia. It is also useful in the long-term treatment of sensory loss, fatigue, urinary incontinence, chills, lower back pain, premature ejaculation, impotence, absentmindedness, memory loss, and chronic kidney and urinary disorders. It is used in Asia to regulate blood pressure. Rehmannia Six Combination can be used for all the same disorders, but is used when heat symptoms are present.

A special note: Individuals with weak digestive function, especially those prone to loose stool, should take a Spleen *qi* tonic such as **Four Major Herbs Combination** along with these Rehmannia-based formulas.

Dendrobium Primal *Yin* Replenisher is designed for people who are dangerously *yin jing* deficient and who show many physical manifestations of degeneration. The formula has a cold energy so that it can quell what are called false fire conditions such as chronic fevers and hot flashes. Even the Rehmannia is the raw variety, which has a very cooling, anti-inflammatory effect. The Dendrobium is extremely effective at replenishing depleted body fluids and *yin jing*. The Tortoise-shell is a profound *yin jing* restorative substance. **Dendrobium Primal *Yin* Replenisher** is not vegetarian. The Tortoiseshell may be removed from the formula, but this will weaken the formula. This formula should only be taken until *yin jing* is restored to a safe level and heat symptoms have ceased. At that time, another restorative formula should be taken that is not so cool, such as **Super Shou Wu Combination** or **Rehmannia Six Combination.**

Essence Restorative is a complete Essence restorative formulation, with herbs that tonify both *yin* and *yang jing*. It is extremely powerful, containing some of the most powerful restorative herbs. It is suited to those people who have burned the candle at both ends for too long. It is capable of rekindling the fire of life. Again, this formula contains Tortoiseshell, but this time as the primary ingredient. It also contains both raw and Prepared Rehmannia so as to completely tonify *jing* while removing false fire. The formula also tonifies *yang jing*. Essence Restorative Formula is especially good for people who suffer from lung weakness and pale, sallow complexion. This is a superb rejuvenation formula for the young or old, male or female, at times of depletion.

Seniors' Programs

As we get older, we need the tonic herbs more and more. As we age, the body does not function as harmoniously within itself and does not harmonize with nature as well either. None of our organs seem to have as much energy as they did when we were younger. By the time we're fifty, almost every organ can use toning up and rebalancing. Frankly, a good diet and exercise program go a long way to reducing the effects of time on our bodies. But the tonic herbs are much more powerful than food at rejuvenating the system.

By now you are aware that Chinese tonic herbalism is an antiaging system which has been developed for the purpose of achieving great longevity. Most of the tonic herbs can slow down aging and prolong life. Many of them are immune system strengtheners that protect us from diseases, be they from external invasion or from our own body attacking itself, as occurs in diseases like arthritis. Many of the herbs protect our vascular system and in particular our heart.

Nothing could be better for seniors than a real tonic herbal program. There is no excuse for degenerating without an effort at rejuvenation. Even if you are suffering from debilitating problems, there is always hope that when the body is provided for, something good might happen. I have seen it happen many times. Sometimes people think that Chinese tonic herbs are miraculous. From one point of view, they are. But from another point of view, they are simply helping the body by providing what it needs but isn't getting.

THE MAJOR CHINESE LONGEVITY HERBS

The tonic herbs are very safe for seniors. Older people have always used the tonics in Asia. They still do—tens of millions of them. Certain herbs and certain formulas have been used so many times that no one is worried about their safety. Here is a list of the most famous Chinese tonic herbs that are really good for all older people.

Polygonum	Deer Antler
Ganoderma	Prepared Rehmannia
Lycium	Schizandra
Ginseng	Astragalus
Gynostemma	Codonopsis
Cordyceps	Eucommia

This list is not by any means exhaustive. Virtually all of the tonic herbs can contribute to longevity and radiant health. The herbs listed here are those most commonly associated specifically with long life in the Orient. Any combination of these will surely contribute to better health, increased vitality, and slower aging.

Certain formulations are especially beneficial to older people. For example, Super Adaptogen contains almost all of these longevity herbs. Here are some other formulas used to increase longevity:

REHMANNIA FORMULATIONS

Rehmannia is a wonderful longevity herb. Many major formulations have been designed around it. The flagship formulation of this genre is called **Rehmannia Eight Combination**, described in detail in chapter 7. It is one of the most widely consumed supplements in the world. Rehmannia Eight Combination is a warm Kidney tonic that tonifies both *yin* and *yang* and disperses stagnant water. It helps regulate sugar metabolism and is thus widely used as a tonic by those with hypoglycemic and diabetic tendencies. It is extremely good for these disorders.

This formula is widely used by senior citizens in China and Japan because it prevents and even reverses many degenerative diseases and disorders associated with the elderly, such as cataracts, urinary incontinence, hypertension, and neuralgia.

This formula strengthens the body and the Spirit and is often miraculous in its results. As always, consult your physician before using herbs if you are suffering from a medical condition.

There is an important variant of this formula known as **Rehmannia Six Combination**. Its effects are almost identical to Rehmannia Eight Combination, but it is more suited to people who have heat conditions. It is thus best for people who have red faces or a bright red tongue and for those who feel hot all the time. Rehmannia Eight Combination contains hot herbs like Aconite and Cinnamon Bark, which warm you up. Rehmannia Six Combination is the same formula minus the warming herbs.

These two formulas are very well known for their health-promoting and healing effects on the prostate gland in older men. They help reduce swelling and inflammation, allowing much easier urination and sometimes vastly improved sex life. Many men have testified to me as to the wonders of these formulas. If one appeals to you, these classics can be obtained at many herb shops or from almost all Chinese health practitioners.

POLYGONUM COMBINATIONS

Historically, Polygonum combinations have been almost always considered to be longevity formulas and highly favored in Asia. Shou Wu Formulation is a premier example of this type of longevity formula.

Though **Hair and Nails Formulation** is named for its ability to promote healthy hair and nails, it could just as easily be called Longevity Formula. Six of the herbs promote longevity, and the other two, Chaenomeles and Notoptergium, have actions that preserve our youth as well. I have my mother on this formula, so you can appreciate how much I like it. She is in excellent health and full of vigor at an advanced age. She has been taking this formula every day for years (two to four capsules each day). She claims that it has brought back her youth. She goes ballroom dancing weekly and enjoys good health. Her hair, which was getting thinner, has completely grown back and is quite healthy. A toenail fungal infection of ten years, which nothing could cure, disappeared soon after she started taking this formula. Her cholesterol has markedly improved. Her neuralgia has almost disappeared. We all think she's getting younger. This is a premium youth-preserving formula.

LYCIUM FORMULA

Lycium Formula is one of the most famous longevity formulas. It is said to have the same action as Lycium but multiplied. It is loaded with longevity herbs and is very safe, like all of the formulas described in this section. It is suitable to men and women, young or old. It is highly preventive and is especially suited for those who want to remain physically active. It is considered to be physically and mentally rejuvenating. This formula strengthens the legs, firms up the back, strengthens all the sense organs, has potent sexual tonic effects, and sharpens the mind. It is said that people who consume this formula every day become cheerful and wise.

GINSENG AND DANG GUI FORMULAS

The formula called **Ten Complete Supertonic Combination** is a superb longevity formula. It is primarily used to build *qi* and blood but has Kidney-tonifying benefits as well. It would most often be used along with one of the prior longevity formulas because they have more influence on the Kidney system (*jing*), whereas this formula has more influence on the Spleen and

Liver systems (*qi* and blood). Ginseng gives you energy. You should definitely take a formula with Ginseng.

REISHI, ASTRAGALUS, AND GYNOSTEMMA

I think it is essential that everyone over fifty consume these three herbs every day. These herbs protect you. They prevent many diseases and they make you healthy all by themselves. They regulate the immune system, make you strong, and keep you smart.

Reishi (Ganoderma) is perhaps the premier longevity herb in the world. It is the veritable symbol of longevity in the Orient. It protects your immune system, your cardiovascular system, your nervous system, your respiratory system, and more. It prevents degenerative disorders and slows down aging. It strengthens your immune system in such a way that it gobbles up bad things before they have a chance to attack your body. As you get older, your immune system weakens considerably. Reishi helps counteract that. Be sure to get the best Reishi you can. Try to find true Duanwood Reishi or wild Reishi. Always use concentrated Reishi, and never the ground mushroom powder that has not been concentrated. Be sure to buy products made from the fruiting body (the "mushroom") and not just the mycelium. The mycelium is nice, but it is not as good as the mushroom.

Gynostemma, which is covered in more detail in chapter 5, is called "Ginseng at a tea price" in China. It is truly great, as it prevents an enormous range of maladies that afflict old people. It gives you lots of energy, but it is not stimulating. It has mild but potent anti-inflammatory action that works all the time to prevent flare-ups. It lowers your cholesterol and improves cardiovascular function. It is a major immune system builder. You may consume it as a tea or take it in capsules. The tea is very good and this is the traditional way of taking it. Remember, it was discovered by the Japanese when they found out that octogenarians were drinking it. It is the rage in Japan, especially among senior citizens. (Japan has the longest average life expectancy in the world. The average woman now lives to be eighty-six years old.)

Astragalus, like Gynostemma and Reishi, does it all. It regulates the immune system and therefore helps protect you against infections. It is an extremely potent antioxidant and therefore has antiaging characteristics. It supports the upright *qi* and therefore gives you the energy to be erect and strong. It helps keep your organs strong and in place, preventing prolapsing and hernias. It fortifies your metabolic and digestive processes and keeps your skin beautiful and healthy. It is a very important longevity herb. Read product labels carefully and be certain to obtain Astragalus that is rich in "total Astragalosides," which are the real active ingredient in Astragalus.

These three herbs are available in one formula, so it is easy to get them all.

CREATING A YOUTH-PRESERVING REGIMEN

If you are really planning on reaching great longevity and staying healthy all the way, like my mother, take a couple of these wonderful longevity formulas every day without fail.

Here's how you create a longevity program for yourself:

1. Choose one of the following formulas described above:
   a. A Rehmannia-based formula
   b. A Polygonum-based formula
   c. A Lycium-based formula
2. Choose a Ginseng-based formula from chapter 7.
3. Take the Supreme Protector formula.
4. Take Gynostemma as a tea or in capsule form.

Take two to six capsules of each formula every day. It is best if you break this into two doses, one in the morning and one at night.

Sexual Tonics

Although Western authorities routinely disclaim any justification to claims that certain foods, herbs, and other substances are sexually strengthening, Asian people scoff at the suggestion that herbs do not influence sex and routinely make use of sexual tonics and aphrodisiacs. Chinese sexual tonics have been found to dramatically improve sexual functioning.

Sexual activity should be a healthful and pleasant experience. However, many people experience disappointment, anxiety, humiliation, and frustration (or even rage) because their sexual functioning is below the standards they believe they should be able to attain. Impotence and frigidity are the cause of great anguish. The Chinese tonics and aphrodisiac herbals have been found through the ages to safely, healthfully, and profoundly fortify sexual functioning, intensifying the pleasure of sexuality and helping eliminate the roots of sexual dysfunction, frustration, and anxiety.

These preparations are not mere sexual *stimulants,* but are great tonics capable of enhancing the health and well-being of those who consume them and are believed by the Chinese and those familiar with Chinese herbalism to help ensure a long and happy life. It is very important to note that the Chinese are not interested in the quick fix when it comes to sexuality. They are interested in building true sexual vitality, and that is the raison d'être for the sexual tonics. Tonics, by definition, are herbal substances that optimize human functioning, improve health, increase longevity, retard aging, are safe even when taken over a long period of time, and have beneficial effects on the psyche. The sexual tonics that come from China meet those qualifications and more.

The herbs are not drugs that alter consciousness like illicit drugs common in the West. But they do relax the body and enable one's feelings to expand. They do strengthen the male genitalia and enhance female sensitivity and response. But it must be emphasized that Chinese sexual tonics are first and foremost designed to improve health.

How the Sexual Tonics Work

Sexual tonics and the sexual Yogas are rooted in the premise that the *jing* can be preserved and even increased. *Jing* has a direct relationship with reproduction and thus with sexuality. *Jing* is regarded as being the root of our existence and is the root of the existence of the species as well. Strong *jing* will generate strong sexual function, while a deficiency of *jing* will result in a weakening of the sexual functions and in the weakening of the body and mind, leading eventually to aging and to death. Thus sexuality and longevity are intimately connected from the Chinese philosophical point of view and in the Chinese way of life. In the Chinese view, it is the goal of all healthful activities to preserve the original *jing,* to replace the *jing* that is spent, and to increase the *jing* that is stored within the body. That is the secret to longevity and to radiant health.

In Chinese herbalism, there are a relatively small number of *jing* tonics, some of which are considered to be *yang* and some of which are considered to be *yin*. The *yang* herbs stimulate the *yang* functions of a human being and the *yin* herbs encourage the *yin* functions. A *yang jing* tonifying herb will cause a man or woman to become more active, more assertive or even aggressive, warmer and more expressive. In addition, the same herbs will cause a man or woman to be more sexually driven and more easily stimulated. A *yin jing* tonic herb will build up hormones, increase sexual fluids in women, and increase sperm production in men. A combination of *yin* and *yang* herbs will both increase longevity and provide very strong sexual energy.

Both *yin* and *yang* are necessary. *Yang* herbs are useless if the reserves of *yin* are depleted. Unfortunately, stress, lack of sleep, overwork, poor diet, chronic or acute illness, and even excessive sexual activity (that is, activity beyond a person's current capacity) can all result in the depletion of *yin* and *yang jing*. Therefore, in building sexual energy in its true sense, one should attempt to regulate one's life so that the causes of *yin* and *yang jing* deficiency are eliminated.

In Chinese sexual herbalism, *yang* herbs are generally not taken unless *yin* herbs are taken also. This prevents the hot, stimulating *yang* herbs from overdriving the system and burning out the *yin* reserves, which are of course required for life itself. But some *yin* herbs can be used alone, although these are generally not as immediately strengthening as a combination of *yin* and *yang* herbs.

THE MAJOR SEXUAL TONIC HERBS

There are a great many herbs used in sexual tonic herbalism, but the major herbs reviewed below are used over and over by almost all Chinese tonic herbalists.

Schizandra is regarded as an excellent *yin* tonic that builds energy in the sexual organs, vastly increasing potency. Schizandra helps to prevent male premature ejaculation. Thus Schizandra increases sexual endurance, allowing a man to engage in intercourse for a much longer time, once he has developed the physical and mental endurance.

Women are also said to benefit greatly from consuming Schizandra. Schizandra is said to increase sexual sensitivity in women and to intensify orgasms. It is considered to be one of the premium women's aphrodisiacs. It is said that after a woman has used Schizandra for one hundred days, she will build up an abundance of sexual fluids. These fluids are stored in the vaginal tissue until sexual excitement causes them to be released. At that time, there is a continuous flow that can continue for an extended period of time. This obviously enhances sexuality and allows her, and her man, to continue for a much longer time (if he has the endurance to stay with her).

Lycium is a major sexual tonic for both men and women and is routinely combined with *yang* herbs in a multitude of formulas used in China. It provides the energy for sex and itself has rejuvenating qualities.

Polygonum is believed to increase male potency and female fertility. Many men report that consumption of this herb noticeably increases sperm production and sexual vigor.

Cornus tonifies the Kidney and Liver and prevents the leakage of sperm. It is considered a powerful aphrodisiac. It generates sexual energy but prevents leakage of *yin jing*. It is thus the perfect sex tonic herb.

Ginseng root is highly prized for its tonic action on the sexual function. Ginseng, which, literally translated, means "man root," enhances both the stimulatory and inhibitory process of the central nervous system, thus improving the adaptability of the nervous responses. It has also been found to increase the production of sex-related hormones and to increase sexual response when consumed in moderate doses. Ginseng has also been found to have profound antifatigue effects and to increase physical stamina. All of these factors make Ginseng one of the most important tonic herbs used in Chinese sexual therapy and Chinese aphrodisiacs.

Deer Antler is perhaps the quintessential sexual tonic. An ancient Chinese classic on the sexual arts states that "there is nothing better than Deer Antler to cause a man to be robust and unaffected by age, not to tire in the bedroom, and not to deteriorate either in energy or in facial coloration." Deer

Antler is a common component of many traditional, and often expensive, elixirs.

Eucommia is beneficial to the Kidneys, the entire endocrine system, the Liver, and the nervous system. It strengthens the middle and lower back, areas that often fatigue or that can be injured during sex. It is widely used in formulas that treat impotence in Chinese medicine.

Epimedium is considered to be the most powerful aphrodisiac herb derived from plant sources. It is famous for its capacity to strengthen the sexual power of men and, in some cases, of women as well. Though it is said to be strengthening to the body as a whole, its remarkable rejuvenating and invigorating effects on the sexual functions is legendary in China. Epimedium, known as "Passionate Goat Herb" in China, increases sexual desire, increases sperm production, and stimulates sensory nerves. The herb has been found to have a moderate androgenlike effect on the testes and prostate. Epimedium reduces blood pressure. It is used in women's tonics as well to increase sex drive.

Cistanche is another important sex tonic that has been used by men throughout Chinese history. Ancient sexual classics claimed that consistent consumption of Cistanche would enlarge the penis. It is also said to make the penis much harder during erections. Cistanche is now known to contain alkaloids that increase blood circulation to the pelvic region in general and to the genitals in particular.

Cnidium Seed, which is in fact Chinese parsley seed, is a sexual stimulant that takes effect very quickly, although not so powerfully as to be overwhelming or uncomfortable. It increases blood circulation to the genital organs and acts as a general catalyst in sexual tonics. Continued intake of Cnidium is believed by the Chinese to make a man extremely potent.

Polygala is used in sexual tonics because it is believed to increase a man's immediate response to female stimulation, while preventing premature leakage of a man's semen. It strengthens the muscles of the back and loins so as to prevent tiring from the exertion and contortions of sexual engagement.

Sea Horse and **Sea Dragon** are powerful *yang* tonics that stimulate the nervous system. Sea Horse and Sea Dragon are superb Kidney tonics which are also renowned in the Orient for their enhancement of the orgasm experience.

Cordyceps is one of the premium Kidney *jing* tonics. Especially when combined with other *yang* herbs such as Epimedium, Cistanche, and Eucommia, Cordyceps is considered to be a first-class tonic to the sexual functions, for both men and women.

Morinda is another *yang* tonic that fortifies the Kidney energy and thus the sexual organs. Morinda is used to strengthen erection, prevent premature ejaculation, help produce sperm, and strengthen the back and knees.

Male Silk Moth is a rare biological agent used in the most powerful sexual tonics. It is regarded in Asia as the ultimate male sexual tonic. Male Silk Moth is hardly ever available in bulk in America, but a number of products are available that utilize this incredible substance.

Dendrobium, or Chinese orchid, is a very good *yin* tonic herb. It has a reputation in the Orient as the "honeymooners' tea." It acquired this descriptive name because it is said to quickly replenish spent sexual energy and fluids, thus allowing for repeat encounters.

Cinnamon Bark is famous for its warming qualities and as a *yang* tonic. When used with other sexual tonics, Cinnamon Bark can greatly enhance their actions, and they in turn enhance Cinnamon's sexual tonic actions as well.

Rehmannia is often used in sexual tonics because it is said to be a superb nutrient to the urogenital system and to enhance the functioning of the Kidneys and adrenal glands, which control sexual function.

SEXUAL TONIC FORMULATIONS

Many formulations have been developed over the centuries that have stood the test of time. These herbal formulations are all safe when used according to standard procedures and with common sense. In fact, they are extremely beneficial. The herbs and formulations are tonics, not medicine or drugs. If you have a distinct medical problem such as high blood pressure, diabetes, significant obesity, kidney or heart disease, or any other medical problem, consult a qualified physician, acupuncturist, or other licensed primary health care provider before taking Chinese herbs. Use your common sense. Don't think that more is necessarily better. It is better to start slowly and allow the tonics to build the system gradually.

Don't use any *yang* tonic herbs if you are sick or suffering from any significant inflammation or from an infection, not even if you have just a common cold or the flu. It is standard practice in Chinese herbalism to refrain from consuming *yang* tonics when you have a fever or an acute infection. Other tonics, such as *qi* and *yin* tonics, are often used to help fight such infections, so these may be used. The tonics described here are traditionally considered to be safe and highly beneficial as health-providing supplements to your daily diet. If you ever think you are experiencing any side effects that are unwanted, discontinue the use of the tonic immediately and either try another formula or consult an expert.

You may use any of the above-described herbs. In addition, you will find many formulas at health food and herb stores that contain these herbs. Here are a few sexual tonic formulas:

Vital *Jing* Formula is a superb *jing* tonic. It is a powerful sexual tonic, suited to any who wish to be highly active sexually. The formula will also generate sexual heat while promoting incredible sexual endurance when taken consistently. This formula may be consumed by both men and women, though it is primarily designed for men. It is a superb longevity and anti-aging formula.

The Emperor's *Jing* was first created for an emperor who had three thousand concubines. It is an extremely potent male-oriented sexual tonic. It is too *yang* for most women. It is the most powerful type of sexual tonic composed of tonic herbs. It is safe for healthy men who wish to increase their potency, or sexual capacity, but should not be used by men who experience hot conditions or by men who lack a ready and willing sexual partner.

Buddha's *Yang* is a vegetarian *yang* tonic that will provide sexual power. It is a hot formula and may require a *yin* tonic to counterbalance its heat.

Many other *yang jing* tonics will increase male sexual power. Some of the formulas described in this book that will have this effect are **Strength Builder, Lycium Formula, Rehmannia Eight Combination,** and **Ron's Endocrine Tonic.**

Beautiful Skin from Within and Without

Perpetually maintaining one's youthful beauty is the desire and target of many men and women. Women in particular consider beauty to be a vital part of their lives, and many work very hard at maintaining beautiful skin. But most people only pay attention to external skin care and overlook the importance of the constitution of the skin. Beautiful skin is maintained and enhanced by nutrients that flow to it through the bloodstream. A healthy internal condition is essential for maintaining one's beauty and preventing rapid aging. When the organs are working harmoniously and efficiently with one another, the body flourishes, and this is reflected in beautiful, radiant skin, lustrous hair, and bright, clear eyes.

Stress, imbalanced diet, inadequate sleep, exhaustion, or anemia may lead to improper nutrition and metabolism by the skin. These factors will promote rapid aging of the skin. All of these conditions have been shown to negatively influence the formation of collagen in the skin, depriving the skin of vitality and radiance—and even accelerating flabbiness and aging of the skin, the formation of wrinkles, cracked lines, roughness, brown aging spots, and black spots. Blood deficiency in particular will lead to rapid aging of the skin, and, unfortunately, many women in America are slightly anemic or do not maintain optimum hemoglobin levels. This results in premature aging.

The Chinese tonic herbs used to promote healthy, beautiful skin provide natural nutrition to the skin. They are effective in enriching the blood with many special nutrients and elements that the skin requires to remain youthful and beautiful. The herbs are superb at moisturizing and nourishing the skin as well as rejuvenating the degenerated elastic and collagen structures of the skin. They can also facilitate blood circulation and metabolism of the skin, functions absolutely essential to maintaining beautiful, youthful skin. And the herbs used in tonic beauty care have powerful antioxidant, free-radical scavenging action that helps remove toxic peroxides from the body and keep the cells youthful. These qualities are essential elements for rejuvenating and maintaining healthy skin, for repairing damaged skin, and for smoothing away wrinkles.

The natural plants and pearls used in Chinese tonic herbalism to promote beauty possess tonic properties. These tonic herbs naturally and safely promote the health of the skin and hair. They have been used in the Orient since ancient times to maintain the youthful beauty of the imperial women. When properly combined and taken over a period of time, they can prevent premature aging and wrinkling of the skin. They can help maintain the moisture in the skin and the skin's youthful smoothness and soft texture. Some of the herbs are blood-regenerating, while others are naturally skin-moisturizing. Still others have detoxifying activity and others have antioxidant and wrinkle-smoothing actions. Centuries of use, as well as recent extensive scientific analysis, has proved that these natural essences have no side effects, which makes them suitable for women and men at all ages. Taking these herbs over an extended period of time can keep the complexion healthy and the skin smooth and firm.

Pearl Powder purifies the skin and makes it radiant. It protects the skin and prevents aging. The components in Pearl Powder help heal blemishes and maintain the health of the skin by participating in its metabolic activities. Pearl promotes the regeneration of new cells and makes the skin smooth, fine, elastic, and naturally beautiful. High-quality Pearl Powder can promote the activities of SOD, the important natural antioxidant enzyme, and can help prevent the development of melanin, which causes freckles and dark patches on the skin. Various components in Pearl participate in DNA and RNA metabolic activities and can promote and accelerate cell renewal, a very important facet of regeneration and beauty maintenance.

It can help prevent the skin becoming old looking, wrinkled, and sagging. This is partly due to its stimulation of SOD activity and partly due to other capacities and nutrients. Consistent use of Pearl Powder can eliminate blemishes such as colored spots and even pimples and boils. Constant use can help assure that the skin will age much more slowly and that it will not be easily harmed by either time or the elements. Pearl is one of the great secrets of the most beautiful women of the Orient.

Pearl is also a powerful antistress supplement. This is an incredibly important effect, since stress can age skin very quickly. It can relieve uneasiness, nervousness, anxiety, and tension. Pearl promotes sound sleep, prevents nervous disorders and nerve weakness, and is commonly used to prevent or overcome fatigue. Consistent use helps a person maintain energy and vitality. Pearl is extremely safe. Safety studies on hydrolyzed

Pearl have shown it to be absolutely harmless. It can be taken by anybody for the course of a lifetime without side effects.

Pearl had always been a very rare and expensive commodity. Until recently, therefore, only the very wealthy could even consider using Pearl as a food supplement to promote their health and beauty. However, over the last decade a new technology has been developed in China whereby pearls are "hydrolyzed." Through modern advanced biochemical technology, Pearl can now be made totally water-soluble. The result is pure "instant" Pearl Powder. The solubility rate of this hydrolyzed Pearl is 98 percent, and of this, studies have shown that 95 percent is absorbed into the bloodstream through the digestive tract. This incredible technological breakthrough has made one of nature's most precious and rare beauty aids available to anyone who wants it. This nearly perfect bioavailability and the enormous reduction in cost makes the hydrolyzed Pearl an extraordinary value.

Not only is Pearl useful for promoting the beauty of the skin, it is extremely useful for women who require calcium, since it is rich in calcium and magnesium.

Ginseng Root is believed to preserve youthful skin. In particular, fresh Ginseng Root is used by women to nourish the skin. Fresh Ginseng is extremely rare in America except in Ginseng products using the new biotechnology Ginseng Cell Culture.

Schizandra is among the most revered beauty tonics. It is said that after consuming Schizandra for a hundred days your skin completely changes. It becomes soft, smooth, and elastic. Schizandra causes the skin to become naturally moist and produces substances that protect the skin from the harmful effects of the sun. It was the favorite beauty tonic of the women of the Forbidden City in ancient Beijing and is one of China's premier antiaging herbs.

Dang Gui is almost always included in beauty formulas because it is the primary herb for enriching the blood and improving blood circulation. It also helps to regulate hormones and slows down aging. All of these factors make it an ideal internal tonic for beautifying the skin. Many skin problems are due to blood deficiency, poor circulation, or hormonal imbalance. This one herb helps with all of these factors. It is especially important if you are under a lot of stress and your skin seems to suffer. Dang Gui is an important herb for women whose skin is sallow, dry, and lifeless—all signs of blood deficiency and hormonal imbalance.

White Peony Root is one of the premier beauty herbs of the Orient. It is famous for giving women pure, silky-smooth skin. It is said in China that "the woman who takes White Peony every day becomes as beautiful as the Peony flower itself." White Peony Root is both a powerful blood tonic, rivaling Dang Gui, and a potent blood-cleansing agent. It removes toxins from the blood by stimulating the liver to thoroughly detoxify the blood. By purifying the blood, White Peony Root purifies the skin.

Longan Fruit is another blood tonic that is famous for beauty. Chinese women consume Longan Fruit to maintain the skin of a young girl—moist, firm, radiant, soft, and smooth.

Astralagus Root, when combined with Dang Gui, improves the circulation of *qi* (vitality) and blood in the flesh. It therefore magnifies the benefits of Dang Gui and all the other herbs in the bloodstream, since it assures that the skin cells will be bathed in purified blood and that all toxins will be removed. Astragalus improves the immune system and helps prevent blemishes from developing.

Lycium Fruit is also famous for making the skin radiant. Lycium is considered an antiaging herb in the Orient. It makes all parts of the body youthful. The skin becomes radiant and firm when you have consumed Lycium Fruit for some time. Recent studies have shown that a group of phytochemicals known as caretenoids have strong antiaging effects on the skin when consumed orally. Lycium is the richest natural source of such caretenoids known. This explains its reputation.

Codonopsis has the ability to balance the primary metabolic functions, to lubricate the lungs, to stimulate blood production, and to make the skin elastic, smooth, and radiant. It is therefore commonly used as a primary herb in beauty tonics.

Ophiopogon and **Asparagus Roots** are superb moistening tonics. These two closely related herbs moisten and nourish the skin, making it soft and radiant. They are essential in dry climates and for those with dry skin.

Dendrobium, the stem of a rare orchid, too is a superb moistening agent. It moisturizes the skin and replenishes fluids throughout the body. It is a famous antiaging herb that, when taken regularly, makes the skin radiant.

Coix is a very nourishing herb that has special effects on the skin. It is famous for its ability to remove blemishes, including aging spots. Recent studies in Japan have shown that Coix can help prevent skin cancer. Constant consumption of this herb makes the skin very healthy.

Sesamum Indicum, black sesame seed, is very nourishing to the skin. It is used in cases of dry, aging skin.

Ginkgo Leaf extract has been shown to improve circulation in the skin and to prevent aging.

Bird's Nest is a powerful and precious *yin* tonic that is very well known in Asia as a beauty-enhancing tonic. It is literally the nest of esculent swifts that inhabit the South China Sea and Southeast Asia. In Thailand, where the best Bird's Nest is found, much of the Bird's Nest is collected by trained monkeys who climb dangerous precipices and into deep caves to get it. It contains a substance called mucin, which is believed to promote the beauty of skin.

BEAUTY FORMULATIONS

Three specific formulations described in chapter 7 were designed to promote beauty and slow down aging from within. **Magu's Secret, Magu's Treasure,** and **Yanlin's Beauty Formula #1** are all superb tonic formulations. Any one of them will contribute to the refinement of the skin, promotion of cell growth and regeneration, and clearing of the complexion.

EXTERNAL APPLICATION OF THE HERBS

Beauty must come from both the inside and the outside. Aging of the skin that is the result of internal causes, such as weak blood, free-radical activity, poor nutrition, toxins, drugs, stress, and worry must be corrected from within. These activities and stress agents make the skin more vulnerable to damage from external causes as well. Dry, lifeless skin will not be able to withstand even a little environmental harshness without further deteriorating. The tonic herbs are the best defense against most negative environmental forces because they build the body's own ability to resist damage and remain healthy.

However, it is also necessary to protect and nourish the skin from the outside, if you want to maintain ultimate beauty. The same tonic herbs, plus a couple of other wonderful natural substances, have the amazing capacity to prevent aging and to protect the skin from environmental damage. Here are some of the substances used by the wealthiest and most beautiful women in the Orient to maintain their youthful beauty.

Fresh Ginseng is one of the most extraordinary skin-beautifying agents anywhere in the world. Since the advent of large Ginseng farms, fresh Ginseng has become much more available. My good friend Ding Jia Yi, a professor at China Pharmaceutical University in Nanjing, is credited with making the modern discovery of the cosmetic use of raw, fresh Ginseng. Professor Ding is the inventor of Ginseng cell culture technology and is one of the most famous and respected scientists in Asia. The story of how he first noticed the effects of fresh Ginseng is known by almost all Chinese since it was described in a newspaper story about fifteen years ago. I asked him to write down the story for me so we could explain his original insight into the use of fresh Ginseng in cosmetics. Here is Professor Ding's story.

It was back in the fall of 1975, I went to the Changbai mountain area to make an on-the-spot investigation on the cultivation and processing of wild medicinal plants such as Ginseng. There I went to a big variety of processing factories and Ginseng-cultivation farms in different areas with different elevations, and a common phenomenon caught my extreme interest. The hands of every worker washing Ginseng was different from those of normal people. Young or old, man or woman, as long as they were Ginseng-washing workers, they had fair, smooth and soft hands. Even older ladies in their sixties had the smooth, soft hands of young girls—although their skin of other parts was in sharp contrast with that of their hands. Seeing this, my first thought was to bring this phenomenon into research so that all the people on the planet longing for beauty could benefit from my discovery and so that everybody could have the hands as beautiful and as youthful as those of Ginseng workers.

At first I did research using *dry* Ginseng material for several years, but the result was never ideal. It was not until I succeeded in cultivating Ginseng cells in large quantities that I was able to create a means of promoting beautiful skin with Ginseng. I was then able to use the active Ginseng cell culture as a main ingredient in a cosmetic. Our natural cosmetics, using this biotechnology, have become a favorite among Chinese women since their appearance on the market several years ago. Usually, the effect of these cosmetics shows after using them for a period of twenty days or so, and using Ginseng cell cleansing cream and Ginseng cell lotion at the same time doubles the effect.

For all this we must thank the soft, smooth hands of Ginseng workers who gave me the inspiration that stirred me into action.

Ginseng Cell Culture Skin Care Products are now available in the United States. Ginseng cell culture technology provides fresh Ginseng cells in their absolute purest form. It is extremely rich in SOD (superoxide dismutase) and related substances. Natural Ginseng-SOD is a powerful antioxidant agent that prevents skin aging. Dried Ginseng and Ginseng extracts contain no SOD. Therefore, creams that contain dried Ginseng or Ginseng extract are not as effective at rejuvenating the skin, whereas Ginseng Cell Culture creams are almost miraculous.

Schizandra phytochemicals protect the skin from the free-radical damage caused by ultraviolet radiation, sunlight. The fruit has an astringent quality that tightens and tones skin, and it helps generate substances in the skin that protect and moisten the skin and help maintain its elasticity.

Pearl powder is used externally to purify the skin, prevent blemishes and age spots, and as a general antiaging agent.

Silk peptides are responsible for the remarkable "silky"-smooth quality of silk. These have now been made available as the result of a biotechnology breakthrough. When applied to the skin, these silk peptides make the skin as smooth as silk, literally! This incredible ingredient is safe and has long-lasting benefits on the skin.

Yanlin's Antiaging Skin-Care Products

The all-natural ingredients include Pearl powder (water soluble), freshly cultured Ginseng cells, and Schizandra extract in various bases. *Ginkgo biloba* extract is added to improve circulation in the skin.

Remember, when it comes to protecting and nourishing your skin from within and from without, "Start young to stay young."

Formulations That Build *Qi* While You Sleep

Some classical formulations have been used for centuries to build *qi* while at the same time helping people to relax, and even to sleep more soundly. These formulations have significant *shen*-stabilizing qualities while simultaneously building *qi* and *jing*.

Ginseng and Zizyphus Combination gets at the root of restlessness and insomnia. It is not a sleeping pill. However, over a relatively short period of time it can prove very effective. Furthermore, you will feel much more energetic during the day. Ginseng and Zizyphus Combination is a major formula for the relief of the type of insomnia where it is difficult to fall asleep. This formula should be used for extended periods of time when treating insomnia. It nourishes *qi* and *yin jing* and stabilizes *shen*, strengthens the Heart, and builds blood. Thus it tonifies all Three Treasures. This formula is specifically suited to those who are experiencing *yin* deficiency, especially if accompanied by irritability, agitation, insomnia, and lack of stability of *shen*.

Ginseng and Zizyphus Combination tonifies Heart *yin*. Heart *yin* deficiency is characterized by mental and emotional instability, absentmindedness, insomnia, heart palpitations, constipation, and sores on the tongue or inside of the mouth.

It has also been used for a lingering fever with no inflammation and a dry red tongue with little coating and a red tip.

Ginseng and Longan Combination is a great *qi* and *shen* tonic formula that has been used for centuries to increase vital energy and calm anxiety. It may be used to strengthen *qi* and blood that have become deficient due to major illness, chronic or acute bleeding, and/or mental or physical stress. It can eliminate insomnia, but in this case the type of insomnia where one has difficulty *staying* asleep. It supports the upright *qi,* helping to keep the internal organs in place. Ginseng and Longan Combination strengthens the immune functions. Some common symptoms for which this formula may be used are anemia, night sweats, absentmindedness, confused thinking, palpitations, impotence, irregular menstruation, prolonged menstrual bleeding, decreased vitality, and chronic fatigue. Ginseng and Longan Combination may be used for pallor, memory loss, and chronic conditions that reappear with an absence of inflammation. It is often used in programs that treat irregular, excessive, or continuous menstruation in weak individuals. Again, this is a tonic formulation, not a drug. It will take a while before its full effects are manifested. However, it is a potent and consistently effective formula.

For Those on an Evolving Spiritual Path

Tonic herbalism was developed to its most profound level under the influence of Daoist and Buddhist masters. These spiritual paths took full advantage of the tonic herbs. Much of the knowledge we have gained has come to us through these traditions. The greatest herbalists in China's history were deeply spiritual men and women, though many certainly had a scientific bent as well.

The Daoists were the great herbal masters. Every Daoist is an expert on the tonic herbs. The Daoist philosophy was deeply naturalistic and featured as a centerpiece the concept that man is one with nature. Many Daoists were hermits and almost all lived in the mountains or countryside. They therefore spent a great deal of time collecting herbs for food and as tonics. The teacher of my teacher, Moo San Do Sha, spent several hours every day collecting herbs, according to my teacher, Sung Jin Park. He and Park would trek through the mountains looking for wild herbs like Reishi, Ginseng, Asparagus Root, and Schizandra. Sung Jin Park told me many stories about how they spent days on end looking for a single special Ginseng root or Reishi mushrooms that would suit their needs. These herbs were treated with absolute reverence. They were holy substances provided by Dao.

All Daoist and Chan (Zen) Buddhist masters knew secret formulas that they used themselves to cultivate certain spiritual qualities and passed on to their disciples. The use of the tonic herbs by spiritual seekers has, in fact, been universal in China, Korea, and Japan for more than two thousand years. They were considered as basic as air. Herbs like Reishi, Ginseng, Asparagus Root, and Schizandra were considered invaluable spiritual substances. Old spiritual texts were full of descriptions of the herbs and how to use them. Ginseng, for example, was described in an ancient Buddhist text as being capable of hastening the burning up of Karma. Asparagus Root, especially the rather rare red variety, was used by the Daoists to open the Heart center. It was said that whoever consumed red Asparagus Root for an extended period of time would become able to fly. Stories abound among the hermits in Korea, where red Asparagus Root is more common, of hermits who lived almost entirely on this nutritious and magical root and actually learned how to fly. Obviously, the metaphor relates to the ability to fly in the spiritual sense.

All of the tonic herbs described in this book fall within the category of spiritual herbs. All are used by Daoists and all can contribute to the development of those who are on a spiritual path. Those who are on such a course should contemplate very deeply the underlying principles of the art of radiant health. They hold the secrets of wisdom and spiritual illumination. The spiritual seeker should be willing to start from the ground up. Start slowly, building *yin* Essence, *qi*, blood, and *shen*. Over time, the focus will shift more and more to building *yang* and *shen*. The effort must always be made to move carefully and to maintain balance at all times. Master Park used to say, "Move slowly, carefully and steadily, and you will soon arrive."

Daoism is considered a "quick" spiritual technique. Many of you will not be particularly interested in Daoism, since you may have your own path. However, the herbs contributed to the "quickness" of the Daoist way. They speed up the process. They harmonize the body, mind, spirit, and nature. They help eliminate toxins and toxic mental conditions. Almost without trying, the herbs can help you grow along the spiritual path. Don't try too hard to master too much of the herbalism at first. You have plenty of time. Consider the herbs a spiritual tool.

Those on the spiritual path should pay special attention to their herbal program. It is essential that the Three Treasures be fully and properly nurtured. *Yin jing* must be fully developed and *qi* must be flourishing. Do whatever you need to do to build *yin jing*. It provides the power for spiritual growth. Then *shen* has the potential to fully expand. There are no specific formulas for *jing* or *qi* for those on a spiritual path. This book is full of such formulas, all of which are of the highest order. Almost any formula provided in this book, or combination of formulas, will do so long as they suit your constitution and where you are in your progress along the path. I do, though, recommend that you seriously consider taking wild herbs as often as possible, particularly herbs like Reishi, Asparagus, Schizandra, and Ginseng. Wild herbs are more expensive. But you should be able to appreciate the difference in a short time. Take a lot of Poria, too. Lycium and Schizandra should be part of your daily program. In any case, always use the highest-grade herbs you can find or afford. Quality makes more difference than any other factor.

Beyond all else, cultivate your Heart. It is the center of *shen*. By all means take Reishi every day and wild Ginseng at least once in a while. Find red Asparagus and eat a piece daily or consume it in a tea.

Shen Tonics and the Spiritual Path

There are two primary types of *shen* tonics: *shen* stabilizers and *shen*-developing herbs. Some of the *shen* tonics perform both functions, although most tend to have one function dominate over the other. Reishi is an example of an herb that does both. Dragon Bone is an example of a pure *shen* stabilizer.

All consciousness, thought, emotions, and passions are under the control of *shen*, which resides in the Heart and which is said by the ancients to be analogous to a central government. These activities are often called unconscious activities because they cannot be directly known or controlled. In effect, they constitute the spiritual part of man, which reflects in his deeds and attitudes to others. The classics say: "When a man is one hundred years old, his organs are empty. *Shen* departs and just the body remains. Life ends."

Hearing, seeing, talking, thinking, working, exercising, are all different functions of *shen*. In health, these activities are performed pleasantly and with rhythm. In sickness, all of these change: there is a lack of brightness, and actions become insane. All these indicate *shen* is being attacked in the Heart. The excessive emotions damage *shen*. Although *jing* and *qi* are ruled by *shen*, if they are wasted (dissipated), *shen* will suffer. This is why moderation is regarded as the supreme way of health, longevity, and true happiness. As Lao Zi said:

The Way is sacred; you cannot own it.
He who would win it would destroy it.
He who would hold it would lose it.
You will find, therefore, that sometimes things
    are in front and sometimes they are behind.
Sometimes there will be strength and sometimes
    there will be weakness.
Thus, the sage avoids extremes, indulgence
    and complacency.

Traditionally, tonic herbs have played an important role in stabilizing and nurturing *shen*. Formulas like **Bupleurum and Dragon Bone Combination** and **Ginseng and Zizyphus Combination** have been widely used by spiritual seekers, particularly at the early stages of their spiritual work. These formulations stabilize *shen* and calm the emotions, allowing *shen* to awaken. Bupleurum and Dragon Bone Combination is still widely used as a meditation formula. It calms the mind without causing drowsiness. It steadies the nerves and soothes the heart.

Peaceful Spirit Formula is an excellent intermediary *shen* tonic that one can use to calm the emotions and build *shen*. Its main ingredient is the Reishi mushroom, the primary *shen* tonic of Chinese tonic herbalism. It is useful for anyone on a spiritual path. It is especially suitable for those who have already made real progress at stabilizing the mind and emotions, but who still slip backward.

Manifest *Shen* Formula is the ultimate *shen* tonic formula, used by intermediate and advanced meditators. It is precisely the kind of formula that has been used by the great Daoist masters, hermits, and sages of the Orient for thousands of years. It is important that the herbs be wild and of the highest quality.

Antistress Formulations

The world is a stressful place. Some people don't have much stress, but I don't know many of these people. To avoid stress, you pretty much have to be a hermit or a true Daoist, living as a recluse away from the world. Relationships, finances, work and career, school, family matters—these and many other factors stress us out constantly.

Stress is highly destructive. If we become too stressed, we do not deal with the stresses appropriately and things often get worse, generating even more stress. In addition, stress is very bad for our health. Many studies have shown that stress depresses our immune systems and shortens our life spans. Stress clearly ages people before their time. It is obvious that we need to know when there is a problem that needs to be dealt with, but that we don't need it to hurt us more than necessary.

Life itself is innately stressful. Virtually any rapid change in one's environment can be defined as a biological stress. Anything that causes the body or mind to have to make a rapid adjustment so as to maintain its integrity is a stress factor. Thus something so simple as a change from daytime warmth to nighttime cold challenges the body's ability to adapt. A healthy person, of course, adapts easily to a wide range of "normal" stress factors. But an overreaction is just as severe as an underreaction. You have to adapt accurately or there will be problems. If for some reason we lose some of our ability to adapt, we will become ill, or at least less than well.

PHYSICAL STRESS

Physical stresses include severe environmental conditions and severe workloads. For this kind of stress, adaptogenic herbs and formulations are appropriate. All of the major adaptogenic formulas like **Adaptogen Energizer, Super Adaptogen, Supreme Protector, Ginseng and Astragalus Combination, Ginseng Nutritive Combination,** and **Ten Complete Supertonic Combination** are excellent. In addition, a well-balanced *jing* tonic such as **Lycium Formula, Shou Wu Formulation,** or **Supreme Creation** is essential to beating stress before it beats you. By taking one or two of these *qi* tonic formulas and an appropriate *jing* tonic formula, we can easily overcome most stressful situations and avoid the repercussions usually associated with heavy physical stress.

These same adaptogenic formulas help us handle stress psychically as well. Our mental and emotional well-being can easily be disrupted by physically stressful circumstances.

MENTAL AND EMOTIONAL STRESS

Mental stress is a different matter. Adaptogenic herbs are still extremely valuable, especially the ones that have a reputation in this area. These include in particular Reishi, Ginseng, Acanthopanax, Lycium, Gynostemma, and Schizandra. Those who are subjected to mental or emotional stress should consume these herbs in abundance. However, it has been found through the centuries that people under severe stress also do very well if they consume *shen*-stabilizing formulations.

Several formulas that have been used for many centuries have regained extraordinary popularity among the heavily stress-burdened in recent years in Asia.

Manifest *Shen* Formula is a premium *shen* tonic with Reishi as its main ingredient, but contains two additional ingredients that make this formula very special: Pearl and Amber. Both of these precious minerals have powerful *shen*-stabilizing qualities which make this formula more suitable for those who are undergoing acute stress and need a supreme *shen* stabilizer that has no side effects, even if taken over a long period of time.

Bupleurum and Dragon Bone Combination is suited to people of strong constitution who are suffering from stress. It is sedating and stabilizing to the mind. It does not cause drowsiness for most people during the waking hours, but simply takes the edge off tension-related nervousness and anxiety. It is used for hypersensitivity of the nerves, palpitations caused by anxiety, chest tension, hypertension, and insomnia due to anxiety. It can be used to establish a calm demeanor by people who become easily frustrated and angry.

Bupleurum Formula is used to inhibit excitability due to an overabundance of Liver *qi*. It is an excellent antistress formulation. It thus sedates the Liver (the nerves), resulting in calmness. It is commonly used to treat irritability, chronic anger, frustration, nervousness, hysteria, tension, spasms, tremors, insomnia due to excitability, grinding of the teeth during sleep, epilepsy, and menopausal disorders. It is superb at relieving "neurotic wry neck," severe neck tension, and spasms due to nervous tension.

Easy *Qi* is a relaxing yet energizing blend of ten Chinese herbs designed to relax, and thus enhance the free flow of energy, especially through the muscles of the back, shoulders, and neck. The formula is based on three great herbs, Bupleurum, Cinnamon Twig, and Pueraria, all of which are renowned in the Orient for their antistress actions. Bupleurum is known for its energy-harmonizing actions. Cinnamon Twig is famous for its circulation-enhancing action and its ability to relax the tension of the upper body. Pueraria is highly regarded for its ability to relax the neck and shoulders and regulate the capillary actions and sinus activity in the head and face. It also contains the Licorice Root/White Peony Root combination that is famous as a muscle relaxer and antispasmodic. Easy *Qi* is the premium example of a Bupleurum-based harmonizing formulation. It is also an excellent digestive tonic.

Help When Traveling

HERBAL JET LAG PROGRAM

When a person travels rapidly across multiple time zones, as occurs when taking a transcontinental or transoceanic flight, the circadian rhythms do not shift at the same rates or in a synchronized manner. This results in poor synchronicity among various body functions and rhythms, resulting in a constellation of symptoms commonly referred to as jet lag. The symptoms of jet lag commonly include insomnia, diminished daytime alertness, fatigue, headache, disorientation, moodiness, diminished cognitive skills, and gastrointestinal distress, including irregularity of bowel movements.

Resynchronization takes place over a number of days, the number of days depending upon the number of transmeridian time zones crossed. Resynchronization generally takes place more quickly after traveling in a westward direction than in an eastward direction. The times of departure and arrival do not have much influence on the circadian rhythms, but the amount of sleep you get while on the plane and directly after arrival does matter. If you sleep poorly on the flight, the sleep deprivation contributes strongly to the disorientation and fatigue associated with jet lag. It has been demonstrated that exposure to afternoon light after a westward flight hastens resynchronization, and exposure to early morning sunlight hastens resynchronization after an eastward flight.

A formulation known as **Poria Five Combination** has been found to be extremely useful for jet lag. By taking this formula every three or four hours starting an hour before the flight and then throughout the flight, jet lag seems to be minimized. You must drink as much good-quality water as possible before, during, and after the flight. This regimen is very good for your health and does not have any side effects.

It is essential that while you are traveling you consume a steady diet of adaptogens such as Ginseng, Gynostemma, Schizandra, Reishi, and Astragalus. Ginseng and Gynostemma provide *qi* and adaptability to handle the stresses associated with the changing environment. They provide endurance and help reestablish natural biorhythms quickly. **Adaptogen Energizer** or **Super Adaptogen**, which contain all of these adaptogenic herbs, are perfect formulas for traveling. I have found that keeping a liquid extract of high-quality Ginseng or Gynostemma with me at all times while traveling can make all the difference in the world. When fatigue starts to set in for no obvious reason, a few squirts of one of these saponin-rich extracts will rekindle your ability to go on.

Gynostemma and Schizandra are both energizing and highly protective. In a new environment, you will be exposed to elements that your body may not be familiar with, including allergens, microbes, toxins, dust, and fumes. Start and finish your day by taking a good dose of protective and self-cleansing herbs like Reishi, Schizandra, and Gynostemma. I would recommend an average adult taking about 1,500 mg of each (three typical capsules) before breakfast and again in the evening. When I am in a dangerous place where there is more chance of becoming poisoned or infected, I double this dose. Take this precaution whenever you enter poor areas of third world countries, whether slum areas or farm country. Obviously, if you visit hospitals or other such areas of possible exposure to dangerous entities, take an extra dose of protective tonic herbs when you get home and for several days following. There are parasites everywhere and it is best to protect yourself to the best of your ability.

Astragalus, Reishi, and Cordyceps are your three primary immune-protective herbs. For this reason, **Supreme Protector**, which is composed of these three herbs, is my choice of protective formulas for traveling. While traveling, never miss a dose. Take extra when your instincts tell you to. In addition, you may want to take a broad-spectrum immune tonic that contains such herbs as Codonopsis, Poria, and Shitake. **Immunity Booster** is one such formula.

If your trip is extensive, be sure to take more *jing* tonics than usual. Traveling can be very stressful, even when it is fun. Whether you are on a ski trip in France or a mercy mission in Central Africa, the body and mind require more *jing, qi,* and *shen*. If your traveling rates as an "adventure," then you need more tonic herbs in general, for sustenance and protection.

Depletion is the cause of a bad ending to a lot of otherwise great trips. Under all circumstances, replenish yourself daily with *yin* tonics. Take extra *yin* herbs like Polygonum, Lycium, Rehmannia, Dendrobium, and Polygonatum. And you will probably do well to take a little bit more *yang* tonic as well to provide the deep energy to do whatever you are doing on this trip. You do not want to exhaust yourself simply because you're having too good a time. You want to come home refreshed and younger from your vacation.

HERBAL PROPHYLAXIS

I always take a couple of mild "medicinal" formulas along with me on trips to exotic places. I usually take **Minor Bupleurum Combination**. It is effective at the first stage of many common infections and is quite prophylactic. In a foreign country, far from your doctor, it is wise to have some protection with you at all times. A formula known as **Pueraria Combination** is also worth obtaining from your herbalist before you leave. It is an excellent formula for the first stages of colds, flus, and bronchitis—diseases people commonly catch while traveling to foreign countries.

You might also pick up an Isatis-based formula to take with

you. It is medicinal, so I won't go into its details here. Just suffice it to say that Isatis is a powerful antimicrobial herb, and a formula based on it is worth having with you in case you get a bad infection and can't find a good doctor.

If you are traveling to outback types of places, a Chinese patent formula known as **Yunnan Baiyao** is mandatory. Don't leave home without it. It is for emergencies that leave you bleeding or with internal injuries. It is a powder that may be applied externally to wounds or taken internally for internal bleeding. It is used to stop bleeding and as a disinfectant. Keep some with you at all times, in your purse or in your pocket. A cut in the countryside in Central America can easily become serious if not treated properly and immediately. Use standard means whenever possible, but you may use Yunnan Baiyao as an adjunct or as an emergency stop-gap. It is amazing stuff.

Vascular Health

The heart and its multitude of tributaries are fundamental to our life. Vascular health is therefore central to becoming radiantly healthy and living a long life. Numerous diseases are associated with the degeneration of the vascular system. Cardiovascular disease is still the biggest killer in America, partly because of the low quality of our typical diet and partly because of ignorance as to how to promote the health of this all-important system.

Many Chinese herbs have been found to benefit the heart and cardiovascular system. Ginseng, Deer Antler, Astragalus, Cordyceps, Reishi, and many others have been proved to maintain the health of the blood vessels in various ways. Formulas containing these herbs include **Adaptogen Energizer**, **Super Adaptogen**, and **Supreme Protector**.

Ginkgo biloba extract is now well known to protect blood vessels. An herb known as Crataegus, or more commonly as

Hawthorn Berry, contains powerful antioxidants that protect the vascular system. The Chinese have been using Crataegus for this purpose for over a thousand years. Many of the Chinese tonic herbs have cholesterol-regulating capacity, Reishi, Notoginseng, and Crataegus being among the more powerful.

It has also been recently reported that as many as 30 percent of all cases of heart failure may be due to chronic inflammatory conditions, which cause ulceration in the large vessels around the heart and ultimately cause severe plaque formation. The immune-modulating herbs are beneficial at building the immune system and mitigating chronic inflammatory responses. Formulas like **Ten Complete Supertonic Combination** and **Supreme Protector** can build the immune system. *Yin jing* tonifying herbs are also very beneficial to the heart. **Rehmannia Six Combination** and **Rehmannia Eight Combination, Essence Restorative, Profound Essence,** and **Dendrobium Primal *Yin* Replenisher** are excellent examples of formulations that tonify *Yin jing* and benefit the heart.

Stress is another cause of heart and vascular disease. Formulas like **Bupleurum and Dragon Bone Combination** have been used for centuries to steady the heart and prevent anxiety-driven palpitations. Peaceful Spirit Formula is also extremely beneficial to the vascular system via its influence over the nervous system.

A formula specifically designed to improve the condition of the heart and vascular system and to maintain its optimal shape is called **Young at Heart**. This formula helps regulate cholesterol, prevents inflammation, improves blood flow, and protects the heart itself. This formula contains all the herbs most commonly recommended to benefit the heart.

Women's Health Issues

Four Things Combination is the primary women's tonic of Chinese herbalism. It is used to regulate the female hormonal system. It has traditionally been used for weakness due to blood deficiency, and pain in the lower abdomen caused by blood stagnation.

Blood stagnation is a condition where the capillaries become blocked and blood cannot flow freely. Women are prone to blood stagnation in the pelvic basin due to the complex arrangement of the reproductive organs in that area. Women frequently constrict the blood vessels in the pelvic basin subconsciously due to any number of psychological or physical stimuli or trauma. From that point on, blood does not flow freely, resulting in blood stagnation. If this stagnation continues over a period of time, blood begins to accumulate and may form clots and pockets of severe occlusion. This is called blood stasis, and is more severe than blood stagnation. Blood stasis can have serious physical and psychological repercussions. Chinese medicine believes that conditions such as ovarian cysts, endometriosis, uterine fibroids, infertility, severe menstrual cramps, and premenstrual syndrome (PMS) are all substantially the result of blood stagnation and/or blood stasis. However, it is clear that blood stagnation and blood stasis may actually result from deep psychological factors that should be handled with *shen* tonics. A blend of *shen* tonics and blood-vitalizing herbs are appropriate for severe stagnation-related problems.

Four Things Combination is used in the Orient for infertility, abdominal pain during pregnancy, blood clots or bleeding after childbirth, menopausal problems, and a deficiency that causes an imbalance of the autonomic nervous system. In addition, Four Things Combination can be used for mild anemia, intestinal, vaginal, or anal bleeding, irregular menstruation, and weakness due to blood loss.

Bupleurum and Dang Gui Combination, known also as Bupleurum Sedative Formula, is a blood, *qi*, and *shen* tonic. It is a classic harmonization formula. This formula vitalizes, smooths, and regulates the flow of *qi* and blood while calming the emotions. It normalizes digestive functions, and it is renowned for its ability to relieve a broad range of female imbalances.

Bupleurum and Dang Gui Combination helps to build, regulate, and strengthen the blood, to relieve Liver stagnancy and congestion, while reducing tension and fire. It helps to cool the blood, eliminating or reducing the tendency of purged Liver toxins to cause surface heat reactions such as headaches, rashes, and hot flashes. Bupleurum and Dang Gui Combination can be used to relieve blood deficiency with the presence of Liver heat, which may result in hot palms and soles of the feet, body aches, a bitter taste in the mouth, dry throat, night sweats, and wiry pulse. This formula has a strong effect on calming the *shen,* helping to reduce emotional volatility, one of the more common symptoms of hormonal imbalance. It helps to calm the central nervous system and is analgesic. It is particularly effective in relieving spasms and cramps in smooth and skeletal muscle.

This great blood tonic formulation can alleviate menstrual irregularities. It is effective in relieving bloating, distension, and aching of the abdomen. It is widely used to relieve many of the symptoms of PMS. Bupleurum and Dang Gui Combination is very effective in relieving menopausal problems characterized by excessive emotionalism and hot flashes. The formula is also effective with such conditions as stress-induced insomnia, decreased appetite, leukorrhea, and convalescence from any illness.

It has a normalizing effect on water metabolism, helping to move moisture and reduce edema, and has a particularly strong effect on relieving bloating caused by sugar intake. It is also effective for reducing the swelling that occurs as a result of tissue regeneration due to an injury, especially where there is a blockage by fibrous tissue, creating a lump. It also helps strengthen and normalize digestive function, improving nutrient absorption.

Bupleurum and Peony Combination is one of the most widely used formulations ever created. It is used primarily by women to regulate their hormones and establish physiological balance. It has the additional function of establishing emotional balance, when hormone irregularities have caused an imbalance. It is used to treat irregular menstruation and many other female problems. Its main greatness lies in its ability to regulate Liver functions and to build blood. Depressed Liver function causes many of the common problems women experience, including PMS and menopausal distress. PMS is caused by a depression of Liver function, so that energy does not flow properly, combined with blood deficiency. This great formulation relieves Liver stagnation, allowing energy to flow freely throughout the body.

This formula is also used for excessive emotionalism, mental instability, irritability, hypochondria, fatigue, and lack of strength. In addition, it dispels fire, which causes feverishness, hot flashes, flushing, and thirst.

Bupleurum and Peony Combination is very effective in reestablishing healthy hormonal balance and menstrual harmony. It can reestablish a regular menstrual cycle within a few months of commencing to use it regularly. It is also used for other common female maladies such as leukorrhea and chronic endometriosis.

In addition to building blood, Bupleurum and Peony Combination warms the Kidneys. By warming the Kidney function, this formula tends to improve female libido and fertility, metabolism, and vitality.

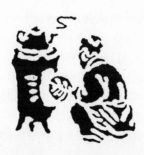

Delivery Systems

COMMERCIALLY AVAILABLE HERBAL PRODUCTS

If you are going to get involved with Chinese tonic herbs, you should know the difference between various "delivery systems." A delivery system is the format in which the product is produced and delivered to you, and ultimately to your bloodstream. There are a large number of delivery systems available, and selecting the right one for you is critical. It is critical for two very good reasons.

First, the delivery system determines the ultimate bioavailability of the herbal components to your system. A delivery system that is appropriate for you is one from which you obtain the highest degree of assimilation with the least stress on your system (hopefully, none).

Second, the delivery system determines in many cases if you will enjoy taking your herbs and therefore continue to take them regularly. It is clear that no matter how excellent a product is, if the person does not take the product as needed, the results are always less than hoped for. If, for example, you hate to take pills because you have trouble swallowing them, it does not matter if the pills are the ultimate substance for your rejuvenation. Eventually, you will stop taking them. Likewise, if you cannot find the time to brew a tonic soup on a regular basis, it is better to take the herbs from a commercial source. Therefore, it is best to find a delivery system that suits your "taste." Fortunately, we are very lucky these days because almost everything you could want comes in a variety of delivery systems.

It is possible to buy over a thousand different Chinese herbs, and with this book you can take full advantage of them. The selection of herbal products that are now available in America is incredible. If you ever visit Asia, there are even more. Hong Kong, for example, has herb shops everywhere, selling thousands of commercially prepared herbal supplements, many of which are tonics. These products are by and large high-grade nutriceutical products made by reputable pharmaceutical or modern-style herb companies.

An herb user has two primary options in using herbs: (1) buy commercially prepared products or (2) buy the raw materials and make your own teas, pills, capsules, or other delivery system. Both approaches have their merits and their drawbacks. But when it is all said and done, if you are serious about tonic herbalism, either approach can get the job done beautifully.

The past decade has seen a virtual explosion in herb companies in the United States. Many of them have become very large, some doing hundreds of millions of dollars in sales each year, and growing. Major pharmaceutical companies are buying into the market now, recognizing that this is a market that is not only exploding now, but appears to be on an endless growth curve. With this rapid industrialization of the herbal industry, quality is going both up and down. Some of the companies are taking advantage of their new buying power by making great purchases and passing them on. Some are investing large amounts of capital in research and development, constantly finding better ways to manufacture the product and maximize the active components. They are investigating the best sources of raw materials by doing sophisticated analyses of the herbs from different places. Many are developing organic farms and are contributing in good ways to third world communities from which they source.

On the other hand are companies that are only taking advantage of the consumer for profit, with little concern for quality. They use low-quality source materials, produce these products cheaply, and dilute them. These companies often spend more money on the label than they do for the herbs in the bottle. Their main interest is in the bottom line.

Most herbs come in a wide variety of qualities. I have already detailed some of the things to watch for. However, with manufactured products, it is going to be difficult to tell what you're really getting. Earlier, I explained that certain herbs reaching this country in bulk are always of good quality, but this only pertains to the herbs that reach the herb shops, particularly Chinese herb shops. There are lower grades of every herb you can imagine. No matter how cheap an herb is, there is always a cheaper batch for sale to a willing buyer somewhere. And usually, it's cheaper for a good reason.

I therefore recommend that you study your sources carefully before you make a big commitment to a product line. Some companies exude authenticity, while others exude slick marketing prowess. The production of herbal products is a true art. It is of course science, too. Making an herbal concentrate, for example, is about the same as making a good wine. You have to know the details of your ingredients and your technology. Batch to batch, herbs change. The technicians have to have a sense for the herbs, a feeling, if they are going to be really good at what they do. Herbal technicians are highly regarded in Asia. They're like fine chefs. It takes years of experience and thousands of batches to really be a master. Most people don't really understand what goes into the production of these herbal extracts. Just know that these people spend their lives watching the details of herbal production, to assure that the product you receive is excellent.

You can consume the herbs in a number of different ways. Herbs these days come in pills, tablets, gel caps, soft caps, and as elixirs, water and alcohol extracts, glycerin extracts, alcoholic *jius* (wines and liquors), pastes, gels, suppositories, tea bags, gum, sublingual sprays, drops, bars, injections, creams, patches, inhalers, etc., etc. In other words, if there's a way to get it into your body, somebody has thought of it and is marketing it at your local health food store, herb shop, or pharmacy.

But again, how do you select a method right for you? Here is some of the basic information concerning various delivery systems.

MODERN DELIVERY SYSTEMS

Concentrated Spray-Dried Powder

Concentrated spray-dried powder is by and large the best form available for most people. The technology for spray-drying herbs was popularized in Japan about twenty years ago. At that time, the Japanese government was establishing its medical herbalism protocol and was setting up strict regulations for production of traditional drugs. Spray-drying technology was clearly the best broad-spectrum technology, and the Japanese government therefore required phytopharmaceuticals to be spray-dried. Taiwanese companies sprouted at the same time. The system has hence spread to China and America. Spray-drying technology is pretty much the standard of the herbal industry in Asia at this time, though it is not the cutting edge.

However, in most cases, it is the most appropriate method for extracting and delivering high-grade tonics as well as medicinal herbal formulations.

Here is how spray-dried herbs are produced. The raw material is first washed and then concentrated in huge tanks, typical tanks holding one or two tons of crude material. These tanks act essentially as large pressure cookers. The extracted liquid is then concentrated and finally dried by the method called spray drying. The resultant powder contains the active constituents of the herbs, but the waste material is discarded and the water is removed. Usually, it will take from five to fifty pounds of crude material to make one pound of finished powder. A product, for example, that takes eight pounds of raw herbal material to make one pound of finished concentrated powder is said to be an 8:1 concentrate. You would have to take eight capsules of the raw material to get the same amount of actual active herbal components as you get in just one capsule of spray-dried powder. Most people prefer to take fewer pills or capsules, and thus compliance was greatly improved with the advent of spray drying.

Spray-dried herbal powders often require a very small amount of excipient in the spray-drying process. Depending upon how sticky an herb is, it will require more or less. Some nonsticky herbs can be manufactured using no excipient. But most individual herbs and herbal formulations require between 3 percent and 10 percent excipient, and some very sticky herbs or formulas require up to 50 percent. A reputable manufacturer will use as little as possible. The most common excipients are cornstarch and microcrystalline cellulose, both of which are natural and easy to digest. Cornstarch is favored in China, and cellulose is favored in America. Some American brands use lactose or other excipients.

Some brands use a small amount of a raw herb, usually one of the ingredients, as an excipient. For example, if a formula consisted of Ginseng, Astragalus, and Licorice Root, the manufacturer might use a small amount of nonconcentrated (raw) Licorice Root powder as the excipient. The raw material is usually irradiated to kill all microorganisms so that there is no chance of contamination. This is pretty much an industry standard for raw materials and is looked upon very favorably by the FDA. The "microbiological" standards for such powders are very strict. Every batch of spray-dried powder is analyzed for such agents as yeast and microbial count as well as for heavy metals, pesticide residues, and other contaminants. Both the Chinese and the U.S. herb industries maintain very high standards regarding these agents, and therefore microbial contamination is very low or nonexistent in herbal products from China at this time. In fact, many Chinese herbs targeted for export are now being grown organically in China.

Spray-dried powders are almost always very easy to digest and absorb, whereas crude drug powders are often difficult to digest. Therefore, absorption in the digestive tract is greatly enhanced by spray drying. This is still the method by which most Japanese, Taiwanese, and high-grade Chinese products are produced. It is the virtual standard of the herb industry. Because the spray-dried powders are generally expected to be better than concentrated herb pills and raw herb pills, the quality of the crude materials going into them is usually much higher, too. The standards established for spray-dried materials are very high and are regulated both by the Chinese government and by market pressures. The competition in the herb business is quite stiff, and most producers use the best commercial-grade herbs they can reasonably obtain to produce the powders, and a few rare companies use better than commercial grade.

Another great advantage of selecting spray-dried powders as your primary delivery system is that by far the greatest number and variety of products are made by this method. There are literally thousands of spray-dried formulations available in the United States. They are produced by large and small manufacturers and are then primarily distributed by herbal practitioners. However, hundreds of formulations can be picked up at major herb shops, and even through distribution systems such as mail-order catalogs and multilevel marketing. In fact, more herbal products are sold through multilevel marketing companies than by any other method. Some of these products are excellent, and some are next to useless. Each manufacturer generally produces several hundred formulas. Most produce the same classical formulations, so as you become more expert you may start to compare companies for quality, freshness, and of course price. Certain brands are always going to be better than others, so study the market a little before you commit to a brand.

At one time, most of the spray-dried powders obtainable in the American market were produced in Taiwan. But many manufacturers have now built or obtained factories in mainland China, and these newer factories are just as good as the factories in Taiwan. The mainland factories have the advantages of experience and expertise, close contact with the actual herb suppliers (not just middlemen), and generally better selection of herbs at favorable prices. Their products are excellent.

The production of concentrated spray-dried powders is a true art. Like making high-quality liquor or real cheese, the technicians involved are true craftsmen and craftswomen. In China, these technicians go through years of university training in the specific craft of extracting and producing herbs. Then it takes years of apprenticeship and experience to become a master herb extractor. Universally, I have found that these people love what they do and they take great pride in the results of their work. A single bad batch can harm people and can ruin a man's or woman's career, so the level of care taken is truly intense. When you receive a capsule and swallow the herbs, you are swallowing more than chopped or cooked herbs—you are consuming the workmanship of a master herbal extractor who has dedicated his or her life to making you healthy and happy.

Most spray-dried concentrated powders are delivered in gelatin capsules. Commonly, these contain between 250 and 500 mg of powder. Most of the top brands are sold this way. Although vegetarian capsules are available, most companies still use bovine capsules, primarily because they are cheaper than the vegetarian capsules. This may be a consideration to vegetarians. But in either case, capsules are easy to digest, they are safe, and they remove the need for binders.

Tablets

Some people like tablets and others find them difficult to swallow or to digest. To some degree, this is dependent on how large the tablet is and what the tablets are made of. Large tablets are difficult for some people; and if not difficult, uncomfortable. Humongous tablets weighing over a gram can be found on market shelves. Generally, however, a tablet of around 500–800 mg, though still pretty large, is comfortable for most people.

You should read the labels on tablet bottles very carefully. Even though most manufacturers have a lot of integrity, tablets are often filled with herbs and excipients that are not really important to your health in the quantities provided. Some tablets are made primarily from spray-dried concentrated powders. These are excellent and of almost equal value to capsules. However, some tablets contain no concentrated material—they are made entirely, or mostly, from ground crude herbs. Remember, it takes many times more of this crude material to equal the weight of the extracted, concentrated powder. In general, for this reason I do not favor tablets made of crude herbs. Most are not potent enough and many are difficult to digest. Far less of the active component is assimilated if the material is crude. Therefore, if the tablet is composed of concentrated herbs, terrific—use them if you like tablets. But if the material is raw, ground, powdered material, you should consider another brand, unless the tablet form provides something you really want and cannot get elsewhere. There are a few excellent brands that use raw herbs in tablet form, but this is rare.

Oral Liquids

A method of delivering the herbs that has been very popular in China for the past two decades is known as the oral liquid, or *koufuye* in Mandarin Chinese (pronounced *ko-foo-yeh*). *Koufuye* are liquid extracts generally sold in 10 cc ampules with a small metal or plastic cap. The cap is quickly removed and the entire oral liquid is consumed in a shot. Usually, a very small straw is provided for delicate consumption. *Koufuye* are sort of the sushi of Chinese tonic herbalism. Almost all of the *koufuye* sold in America are tonic formulations. Each one contains at least one famous or specialty supertonic, and in some products more than one. The oral liquids are usually water extracts, though some are extracted with alcohol and water. Since they are bottled in individual doses, spoilage after opening is not an issue. They are bottled in special machinery that prevents microbes from entering, and therefore they can last for years if left unopened and stored in a cool, dark place. Most are sweetened with honey to make them easily consumable. In fact, most are quite pleasant. Some of the *koufuye* that have been on the market are absolutely superb products.

Koufuye are ubiquitous in China. Almost every herbal factory has a *koufoye* "workshop" (division), and if it doesn't, it can hardly be considered a real nutriceutical factory. The most famous *koufuye* are known all over the world. Some, like **Peking Royal Jelly** and **Panax Ginseng Extractum**, in its familiar green box, have been available in most health food stores throughout the world for almost twenty years. However, these are hardly even worthy of being called the tip of the iceberg.

There are over a thousand *koufuye* in China, of which about twenty are routinely exported to America.

Water Extracts

Water extraction is probably the most common traditional method of herbal extraction. Many products are still extracted with water, but water extracts do not last long naturally. Refrigeration can preserve a water extract for a few days, or even weeks, but this is not sufficient to allow for commercial production. In order to create a commercial product for the mass market, modern preservative methods are required. The recent development of natural preservatives and preservation technology has made this method of delivery more popular.

There is one absolutely great way to obtain liquid extracts commercially. Some professional herbalists now have their own professional extraction units. They can therefore prepare water, or even alcohol, extracts of the tonic herbs on a custom basis. This is absolutely ideal. If you can find a good herbalist who provides such a service, you are in great shape. These extractors can prepare up to a month's supply of pure herbal tea, each dose individually packaged in an FDA-approved retort package, which precludes the need for a preservative. Frankly, this method is awesome. If your herbalist has such an extractor, uses premium-grade herbs, and has a good understanding of the principles of the Superior Herbalism, it is almost impossible to do better.

Herbal Liquor

There is another form of liquid extract that is both ancient and extremely popular in Asia—"herbal liquors." In Chinese they are called *jius*. There are hundreds of these herbal liquors in

China. Every grocery and department store has a section devoted to them. In fact, in many areas the herbal liquor section will contain more products than the regular liquor department. Most of these herbal liquors have a fairly high alcohol content because it helps ensure the preservation of the herbs. Though the tonics are often called tonic wine, they are generally much more potent than the beverage we normally call wine. The alcohol content of these drinks usually ranges between 30 percent and 50 percent alcohol. They are more like vodka.

Unfortunately, Chinese tonic wines are generally not available in the United States due to importation restrictions. However, if you can drink alcohol and if you ever visit China, Taiwan, Korea, or Hong Kong, by all means buy a few bottles and bring them back for personal use.

The recommended way to consume these tonics is to take one or two shots each day, usually after dinner or at bedtime. The alcohol aids in the rapid assimilation of the herbs and there is very little waste. Alcohol tonics tend to work quickly. They are very efficient for extraction, so they make the use of very expensive herbs like Deer Antler, Cordyceps, and premium Ginseng more economical.

Tinctures

There are many brands of herbal tinctures available in America. Virtually every natural food store in America carries a selection of tinctures, and some of the major stores carry dozens or even hundreds, many of which are made of Chinese herbs. These tinctures are concentrated alcohol extracts. They provide the alcohol-extractable component of each of the herbs included in the formula. Some of these are very fine products, while others are weak. Most are delivered in one- or two-ounce apothecary bottles with a dropper. Usual doses range from ten to thirty drops, or one to three squirts of extract each time, two or three times daily.

And when it comes to quality, as always, the company makes all the difference. Select your tinctures well, by brand, by product, and by concentration. Then judge by taste, feel, and effect. I would tend to select the tinctures made by companies that specialize in Chinese tonic herbs. The companies that produce a very wide range of tinctures from around the world tend to know much more about American, Latin American, Native American, and European herbs than they do about Asian herbs. Asian herbs generally require a company's full attention if quality is going to be *really* good.

Concentrated Hydroalcoholic Extracts

Some producers make highly concentrated extracts that are produced with both water and alcohol. These are the best of the commercial "tinctures." These can be extraordinary if the herbs used are high-grade. These extracts contain all of the active components of the herbs because almost all active biological components will be extracted by alcohol or water. The way to judge these is simple: the product should be highly concentrated and should be made from premium herbs.

These extracts are measured according to how much raw material it takes to produce one gallon of the concentrated liquid. If it takes one pound of herbs to make one gallon of finished extract, the concentration is said to be 1:1. If it takes eight pounds of raw material to make one gallon, the concentration is 8:1. Obviously, an 8:1 concentrate will contain much more material than a 1:1 concentrate. An 8:1 concentrate will tend to be thick and startlingly tasteful. Concentrates this high are extremely rare in the marketplace because they cost much more to produce than lower concentrations. Most companies feel that the consumer cannot recognize the difference between a 2:1 and an 8:1 concentrate. But this is a financial excuse. The fact is, users recognize the difference immediately, and even more so as time goes by. Concentrates of 8:1 are primarily made by specialty shops. These shops will charge more, but that's because they are using much more raw material. Moreover, they generally tend to use much higher-grade herbs. Note that some products cannot be concentrated to an 8:1 ratio. Premium Deer Antler, for example, turns to paste if concentrated above a 4:1 ratio. Even at 4:1, Deer Antler is very thick and in cold weather will tend to gel up. However, most Deer Antler products are much less than 4:1. In fact, most are more like ½:1 or even more diluted.

In addition, an 8:1 concentrate from one company may be very different from that of another company. The lesser-quality company will select lower-grade herbs and the resulting product will be thinner and will not taste as good. Secondly, the method of extraction is a true art. There are many tricks to extracting herbs. For example, if the herbs are not chopped well, the resulting extraction will be much weaker than that produced by someone who thoroughly chops the raw materials. Unfortunately, the ultimate decision can only be made after you have sampled the product, tasting and experiencing it.

In selecting tinctures, be sure that you are getting the herbs that you want or need. Specialty shops have more complex formulations, whereas natural food stores tend to have simpler products. But without question, it is possible to obtain fabulous products at either type of venue, and it is equally possible to make mistakes at either type. Ask questions and know what answers you need to hear.

Tea Bags

A few superb formulations require infusion rather than decoction to extract. In other words, for these particular formulations, steeping is appropriate rather than boiling. But frankly, there are very few of these products. Most Chinese herbs require extended decocting (simmering) or extracting in alcohol. However, green leafy materials and flowers generally lend themselves to delivery via tea bag. One prime example is tea. Everybody knows that tea only needs a short period of steeping to extract its active ingredients, including its caffeine and its all-important polyphenols. Another major example is Gynostemma. The active components of Gynostemma are in the leaf. Therefore, Gynostemma is frequently provided in tea bags. A few minutes of steeping Gynostemma yields a potent herbal tea worthy of the title "supertonic."

The Chinese are masters of the so-called medicated tea. These teas use tea leaves as a carrier, or delivery system. Other herbs are decocted until they are highly concentrated. The tea leaves are soaked in this concentrated liquid and dried. The herbs are absorbed into the tea leaves. When you steep this medicated tea, the extract is released into the water along with the active ingredients of the tea leaves. This can produce a potent drink. Most medicated teas in China are used to deliver medicines, especially cold and flu medicines, although a few brands of tonic teas are prepared in this manner.

A twist on this method is the use of Gynostemma as the tea base. There could be no "tea" better than Gynostemma with various tonic herbs soaked into it, ready to be released when the Gynostemma is put into hot water. The ultimate example of this is the product known as **Spring Dragon Tea**™, which is composed of Gynostemma as the base and various adpatogenic herbs in concentrated form soaked in. The concentrated herbs are Acanthopanax, Lycium, Schizandra, Astragalus, and Lohanguo.

PREPARING THE HERBS YOURSELF

There is nothing like preparing your own herbal tonic. I firmly believe that everyone should try it sometime. Once upon a time, everyone prepared their own teas, pills, and wines. But that was in another era. Today, few people have either the time or the motivation to boil a new concoction every day. However, I cannot emphasize too much that you should make a tea at least once, just to get a feel for what the process is. Some of you will really enjoy it and can continue to make teas throughout your lifetime. If you master this art, you have mastered something truly great.

By making your own teas or herbal liquors, you have the opportunity to control every herb in the mixture. You get to select the herbs, decide how much of each one you want to include in the formulation, and you can control the process of preparation. When you finally consume the product, if you did a good job, the tea or liquor will be especially appreciated. Here are tips on how to prepare the Chinese tonic herbs in your own kitchen.

Preparing Herbal Brew

Extracting the Chinese tonic herbs in water generally requires simmering for some time, until a specified concentration is achieved. This process is known as decocting. Traditionally, herbs were usually prepared either in a clay pot or double-boiled in a "ginseng cooker."

COOKING IN A GLASS, PORCELAIN, ENAMELWARE, OR CLAY POT

Prepare a formulation from the raw materials by placing the herbs on a plate. Place the herbs in a mesh strainer and wash them under running water to remove all the dirt that may be present. (Chinese herbs sold in herb shops have in most cases already been carefully washed.) There are a couple of herbs you should *not* wash. In particular, do not wash Ganoderma (Reishi) if it is covered with spores. The spores will wash away. The spores are a critical and valuable component of the herb.

Place the washed herbs in a porcelain, glass, or clay pot. Always use premium-quality herbs for home brewing. Do not use a metal pot, as the metal is believed to react with herbs like Ginseng, making them much less effective. Iron, copper, and aluminum pots are the worst. Stainless steel is probably not very reactive with the herbs, but still, I have to advise against it. Porcelain, glass, and clay pots are inert and are perfect for cooking herbs. Crocks work well, too. Some people say that you should not use enamelware pots. But I have never understood why not. In fact, I used a trusty enamelware pot for fifteen years. I used it only for my tonic cooking. I didn't cook anything else in it. Finally, some of the enamel chipped away, leaving a small patch of the underlying iron exposed. Hence, I have retired my beloved enamelware herb pot.

Traditional, inexpensive, Chinese clay herb pots may be purchased at Chinese markets. But they are cheaply made and crack in short order. In fact, before you purchase one, have the shop owner fill the pot with water to see if it leaks—a high percentage do. I consider them a novelty, especially when you compare them to the great pots that you can buy these days. My recommendation is one of the following: a great enamelware pot, a Pyrex-style glass pot, a porcelain pot suited to stovetop cooking, or a Crock with a clay inner pot. I have used them all and they all work wonderfully.

Add pure spring water to the pot. I like water that has been purified and yet is rich in trace minerals. I own a special apparatus that I obtained in China that naturally mineralizes water.

Alternatively, I sometimes add a couple of teaspoons of Great Salt Lake liquid mineral concentrate to the tea water. It changes the flavor somewhat, but it adds over eighty trace minerals, and my body and mind appreciate that. Alkaline water is best for your body.

The rules concerning the amount of water you use are really just relative. People say all kinds of things and make all kinds of recommendations, but in reality, it is a matter of personal taste. You may add as much or as little water as you like. If you add very little water and cook for a long time, it may boil away. If it doesn't boil away, it will be extremely potent. If you add a lot of water, the resulting tea may be weaker. But I have found through my own experience that it is okay, or even better, to use plenty of water. If you use premium herbs, the tea will still be very potent. Often, people make their teas too strong and their bodies are overwhelmed by the effect of the herbs. I like my teas rich but palatable. Moderation in all things—that's my motto.

Bring the brew to a boil. Watch carefully so that the tea does not boil too hard. If it boils too violently, even for just a minute, it will damage many of the constituents of the herbs. As soon as it reaches a boil, turn the heat down so that the tea simmers gently. Most of the tonic herbs should be simmered for at least one hour, and preferably two hours. Aromatic herbs rich in essential oils like Ligusticum and Cinnamon Bark should only be cooked for a short time, however. Ligusticum and Schizandra, for example, should not be cooked for more than fifteen minutes and Cinnamon Bark for not more than five minutes. Therefore, you will want to add these to the brew at the appropriate time in the cooking process.

I advise you to have a timer close to you. You do not want to forget about your tea because you have become involved in a ball game on the TV or in a telephone call. I admit that more than once in my life I have forgotten a tea on the stove and burned the herbs and ruined the pot. In each of these cases I wasted very expensive Ginseng roots and other valuable herbs. I am not proud of it, but it taught me to set my own biological timer. In addition, I have a timer on my desk which I set when I'm making a tea to remind me of the different steps. I have not wasted a tea now in many years (not since I turned $300 of premium Korean Heaven Grade 15 Ginseng roots into charcoal).

When the brew is done, let it cool down a bit and pour yourself a cup. Enjoy your work and with each sip taste the antiaging and *shen*-building factors in your awesome tonic tea. Let the brew cool naturally for about half an hour, then strain it. If you plan to reuse the herbs, put them in a container and put it in the refrigerator or the freezer. Be sure to refrigerate the rest of the tea at this time. Leaving a tonic brew out for a little too long will cause it to spoil. These tonic teas are very rich and they will spoil quickly. Each time you want a cup of the tonic, pour a cup and reheat it, but put the rest back in the refrigerator immediately. Make it a rule to never let a tea spoil or go to waste. It's a matter of respect. And drink each batch to the bottom. Drink all such teas within one week. They may last considerably longer in the refrigerator, but this one-week limit is insurance. If you want, you may consume the tea more quickly. You will have to be the judge as to how much to drink and how often. Depending on how strong the original herbs were and how potent you made the brew, you will adjust the amount you drink accordingly.

Tonic brews generally taste quite pleasant. Most are naturally sweet. However, they will all be strong-tasting and may require some getting used to. If you need to, add a little honey or liquid Stevia extract. I never do, but many good herbal people do. So don't feel embarrassed if you do. But the next time, you may want to add a little more Licorice Root, Jujube Date, Longan, or Lohanguo. All these herbs contribute both to the tonic and to the taste.

COOKING IN A "GINSENG COOKER"

A ginseng cooker is a Chinese porcelain cooking pot made especially for cooking small batches of expensive tonic herbs—and particularly for cooking expensive Ginseng roots. The typical ginseng cooker is small. Even the biggest ones are not large. They have two lids to ensure that the steam stays inside the pot. Here's how you use a ginseng cooker.

Place the herbs in the cooker. Do not put too much material inside the cooker. They are made for a little bit of something very special. Add water to within an inch of the top. Replace both lids. Put the cooker into a larger pot. Fill the larger pot with enough water to cover at least two-thirds of the ginseng cooker.

Turn on the heat and bring the water in the outer pot to a boil. Turn the heat down so the water simmers. Watch carefully that more than half the water does not boil away (and certainly not *all* of the water, God forbid—you'll burn down the house). Add water occasionally. I have developed my own technique here. I always put hot tap water into the outer pot to replenish it. This way, the ginseng cooker and the tea inside it are not shocked by a sudden lowering of temperature. It quickly resumes its simmer and the tea inside the cooker hardly knows there was a water change.

Continue cooking like this for two to six hours. Turn off the heat and, with a towel or pot holder, remove the ginseng cooker. When you remove the lids, you will notice that none of the inner liquid has been lost. The liquid in the ginseng cooker never quite reached boiling. The double lid recycled the steam. This tea is extraordinarily rich. Strain the herbs and save them if you want. Drink the tea within a short time.

Ginseng cookers are the best way to cook Ginseng, Cordyceps, Bird's Nest, Deer Antler, and other very expensive, premium tonic herbs.

Cooking in an Electric Herb Pot

In the past few years, electric herb pots have popped onto the scene. They are designed specifically for cooking Chinese herbs. They have either a clay or a glass pot and an electric timer. They also control the temperature. Mine has two temperatures, one that generates a hard boil and one that generates a simmer. I set it for hard boil until it comes to a boil, then I switch to simmer.

I really like my electric herb cooker. Now that my trusty enamelware pot has boiled its last Codonopsis Root, I have switched full-time to my new electric pot. It does a perfect job every time. I put in the herbal formula and fill the pot with good water. I set it to two hours (the maximum allowed on my unit). The only steps I have to perform are to turn the heat down once it hits boil and to add herbs like Schizandra, Ligusticum, and Cinnamon Bark at their appropriate times near the end of the cooking. Therefore, I still use my timer and keep it where I'm working (or snoozing).

Like the other procedures, when it is done, strain the tea and put the herbs away if you choose to do so. Refrigerate the tea and keep it refrigerated until it has been entirely consumed.

I think that all serious herb users should have either a beloved herb pot that they use only for their herbs, or an electric herb pot from either China or Korea. It's a small commitment to your perpetual use of the extraordinary Chinese tonic herbs.

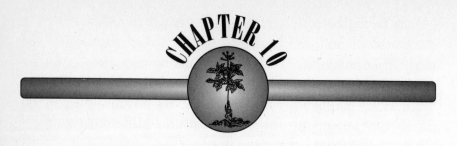

Six Lessons the Tonic Herbs Have Taught Me

Late one night I was contemplating the meaning of life and it came to me that the herbs with which I have been involved for so many years have taught me some of the deep truths of life.

As soon as I started consuming Chinese tonic herbs, my life virtually turned around. Within a matter of days, I recovered much of my energy, and though it took some years to fully regain my health, I felt vital and strong within a month. The original herbal formulas were simple by my current standards, but I feel that they saved my life.

It is said in the East that for a person to truly develop, he or she must suffer one great disease. This "disease" might not be an actual sickness—it can be anything that deeply challenges us to overcome our prejudices, our weaknesses, our fear, and our ignorance. As a result of my struggle to regain my health, I had a realization that when a person has already become ill, the curing of the disease can often be delayed by the person's attitudes. The lessons contained in his or her afflictions have not been absorbed, and upon recovery, he or she will immediately plunge back into the ways that caused the original sickness. For this reason, it is imperative that the spiritual aspect of a person (*shen*) be considered in all human dysfunction and that the emotions and desires that block the full expression of the true self be moderated or eliminated.

The sickness I suffered forced me to face myself and to grow. Quite wonderfully, I discovered that, in their great wisdom, the people of Asia had long ago developed a system that could help a person such as myself move through such challenges so as to attain health, happiness, and some degree of wisdom.

Amazed at the potency of the tonic herbs, I spent the next several years seeking out teachers who could instruct me in the ways of herbalism. Because the herbs that seemed to save me were Chinese, I sought Oriental masters who could teach me their ancient knowledge and allow me to penetrate the secrets inherent in the system. There were no schools of Chinese medicine in America in those days and herbs were not readily available yet, so I had to find teachers in the Asian communities who were practicing essentially underground. I was an enthusiastic student in those days, and I found a number of excellent teachers, most of whom were Chinese. The Chinese teachers I met at that time tended to be very practical but did not want to go deeply into the principles underlying the practicality. A Korean teacher, Sae Han Kim, was the first teacher who really got into how the herbs worked and into their subtler applications.

Ultimately, I met my teacher, Sung Jin Park, and he taught me the details of the Daoist art of radiant health. I helped Master Park translate a number of manuscripts as he helped me to understand the principles of the human energy system, the laws of nature, the basics of Superior Herbalism, Daoist breathing techniques, Daoist exercises, and a few other things. He was a great teacher to me. He had a way of communicating to me extremely subtle ideas that nobody else could explain. He used few words, but his expression was pure wisdom. Then, one day, he returned to Korea to live as a hermit in the mountains with Grand Master Mu San Do Sha, his teacher. I have not seen him since.

Master Sung Jin Park took me deep into the realm of tonic herbalism. He emphasized the attainment of radiant health rather than the eradication of disease factors. This emphasis on health promotion was a major turning point in my life. Up until that time, I had primarily relied on the Western model of health care, which emphasizes remedial care "after the fact." As my training proceeded, Master Park instructed me never to become a "healer." He said that "healing" in the general sense is always temporary. He told me to become a teacher, or in his words "an agent of *shen*" ("the light-bearer"), who guides people in their transformative processes, so that *many* could benefit from this knowledge.

When it came to herbal training, Sung Jin Park taught me only about the tonic herbs, almost completely ignoring medicinal substances. He believed that radiant health could be achieved by anyone with the will to achieve it and that the tonic herbs were the principal component needed to achieve radiant health, even if problems exist that appear to require medicine. He also believed that *qi gong* and meditation were necessary if one was to achieve the pinnacle of radiant health. He helped me overcome a number of medical problems without ever giving me a medicinal herb. We met several times a week, and each time he would recommend a formula that I would then prepare and drink over the next couple of days. My health improved radically during the time that I was under his training.

Master Park left me before I learned all the details of each of the tonic herbs themselves. The incredibly subtle details of such an art can only be learned by experience over a long period of time. I have spent the past two decades making the tonic herbs part of my daily life and introducing them to as many others as I possibly could. I made a commitment to Master Park that I would train others in the art of radiant health, and have done all in my power to keep this commitment. In many ways, the herbs have become my teacher, and there are six lessons that I have learned from them.

1. Faith in Nature

We have evolved over a period of millions of years, by design or otherwise, into true superbeings. Nature is so vast and mysterious. No one will ever understand all its subtle and intricate nuances. But its basic laws are clear. Nature nourishes those that live in close harmony with it and destroys those that move too far astray. If we destroy our environment, we will eventually perish. This law applies to our internal being as well. Modern medicine has brought forth many miracles. Yet maintaining our health is the responsibility not of "medicine" but of our own knowledge of how to live as nature means us to live.

Chinese tonic herbalism is based on the premise that it is possible to attain a state of health known as radiant health, which is defined as "health beyond danger." The simple idea is that it is best to build a powerful and healthy system rather than wait until disharmony and illness set in. I do not believe that anyone can argue with this concept. Certain Chinese herbs have come to be revered because they seem to be profound health aids (not "medicine"), and have been found over many centuries to be extremely safe when used moderately and appropriately. These are the superior herbs.

These herbs seem to help us attain and maintain an organic and psychic balance even under stressful conditions. The Chinese tonic herbs have taught me to have faith first in nature and then in the nature that resides within me, since I am one with all of nature.

More recently, I have learned that the best things come from nature. With the advent of the phytonutrient revolution, it is becoming more and more clear that the most powerful and wonderful treasures relating to our health and happiness are all natural. Synthetic and artificial foods and supplements cannot hold a candle to the bounty of nature's own supernutrients. Science is confirming what Chinese herbalists have been saying all along—the laboratory cannot match nature.

2. Patience

Even though my illness seemed to reverse itself abruptly, it took me many years to become what I believe to be truly healthy. And I came to realize that maintaining my health is a moment-to-moment exercise in life. Health is more than just freedom from disease, although that certainly is a minimal requirement. Health is actually a state of vitality that allows us to fulfill our greatest destiny while we are alive on this planet. It is a vitality that allows us to adapt optimally to the many changes we go through daily and over time, without becoming exhausted, without using up the precious reserves that sustain our lives.

We all may continue to grow on the spiritual plane for as long as we exist. Growth is fraught with danger, failure, and struggle. We must overcome many hardships, and we must overcome ourselves continuously. It is the art of overcoming difficulties that allows one to grow and become the most that one can become. The greatest failure is the inability to overcome the challenges that are required for true human growth. I have learned that the tonic herbs are an almost miraculous tool for a person on a serious growth path. They provide the power and adaptability required to survive the downtimes. I feel that they have helped me develop my power of will and the creative capacities that have allowed me to find ways around the obstacles that have blocked my path. And the tonic herbs provide protection, stability, and creative vitality during my strong times, allowing me to grow.

The tonic herbs help us to become emotionally strong, calm, and adaptive and to understand the big picture of life. They have helped me to become patient. By being patient, I have learned how to avoid exhaustion, and by being patient, I have learned that one can attain almost anything that nature allows for us as human beings.

3. Self-Respect

By taking tonic herbs that are harmless and yet so incredibly nourishing in so many ways, I have come to respect my own body, mind, and spirit. I have learned that junk food, abusive and harsh behavior, offensive chemical substances, and the like are self-destructive and self-deprecating. I have learned that it is essential to respect oneself deeply if one is to attain any level of health and happiness. I have come to know that I have, like every other human being, a higher purpose that can only be attained if we have self-respect of the highest order.

Furthermore, by respecting oneself, it is possible to respect others and to respect nature and all its manifestations, both animate and inanimate. I have observed a deep lack of respect among people in our society, and this will not be corrected with money or academic education or medicine. It will be corrected when we have true self-respect and realize that we are all great and that we are all one. Self-respect therefore extends to everybody and everything in human society and in nature.

4. The Value of a Positive Attitude

Chinese tonic herbalism is based upon the premise that by taking certain very healthy substances we can attain a very positive healthy state. With a strong immune system, a strong vascular system, a strong mind, a strong structure, and a strong nervous system, we will avoid or be able to overcome most dangers and we might even live longer, better lives. This makes sense to me. If we spend all our time concentrating on our weaknesses and problems, we will never cease putting out fires, since our attitude is awry. I am not saying that one should ignore a problem. That would be foolish. There is the Oriental saying, "When a problem is acute, treat the stem; when a problem is chronic, treat the root." After dealing with the problem, and even during that process, continue to focus on creating positive health.

As a general principle for living and acting, emphasis should be placed on creating well-being and positive achievements. The tonic herbs tend to generate that attitude and are in this sense very positive.

5. The Meaning of "Moderation"

"All things in moderation." These are words of wisdom that we have all heard but by which few abide. Excessive behavior, including all compulsive and/or addictive behavior patterns, destroys our ability to live naturally. And though we live in unnatural environments, we are still natural beings under the influences of the sun, the moon, the stars, gravity, the weather, the air, our food, water, and the earth.

Excessive behavior imbalances us and drains our energy. Excessive behavior inevitably and invariably results in disharmony. Excessive activity drains our energy and our energy reserves. Excess in any aspect of our lives can be dangerous and will inevitably lead to trouble and possibly catastrophe. Thus the saying in Chinese tonic herbalism that "it is all right to become fatigued, but never to become exhausted." Fatigue is natural and even healthy. However, exhaustion means that we have drained ourselves, going beyond our normal limits, depleting energy reserves. Such depletion is much harder to recover from than mere fatigue. In fact, many people never do recover from a bout of deep exhaustion.

Again, as the great Zhuang Zi once wrote,

> When the shoe fits, the foot is forgotten.
> When the belt fits, the belly is forgotten.
> And when the Heart is right,
> "For" and "against" are forgotten.

The great wisdom expressed in this proverb can only be experienced and appreciated when we have attained a dynamic balance and harmony with nature. The great Chinese tonic herbs are some of nature's sublime gifts. They can help the "shoe to fit," they can help the "belt to fit," and ultimately and most important, they can help the heart become "right," allowing us to rise above the illusionary world of duality and to know nature as it is, as a complete, unified, harmonious being, of which we are a part.

The tonic herbs can help restore that balance, harmony, and energy and are themselves the very essence of moderation. They can also help us sense our limits, to maintain our center, and to have the strength and wisdom to stop when we need to.

6. Love *Is* Everything

As we learn the other five lessons over time, we come to experience a sense of profound love for life, for nature, for ourselves, for our earth and all its beings, for humankind as a whole, and for all the members of our human family. Love is the ultimate truth. Love really is everything. And indeed, everything is love.

Our true Spirit, which the Chinese call *shen,* is the spark of divinity that resides within the heart of every human being. *Shen* is the guiding light by which all of us are capable of growing toward illumination. All beings possess *shen,* including animals and plants, which are generally abundant in *shen.* Even many minerals possess *shen* in crystallized form. Mountains possess *shen,* as do all aspects of nature. But it is in the human being that *shen* comes to full expression.

Shen resides in the heart and manifests as love, kindness, compassion, generosity, giving, tolerance, forgiveness, mercy, tenderness, and the appreciation of beauty. It is the Spirit of a human being as the divine messenger, the channel of God's will and love. *Shen* is the purpose of all spiritual paths. It is Buddha's desire to end suffering and it is Christ's love and compassion.

Generally, though, this light, this love, is buried in the heart of a human being, hidden behind a thick, opaque layer of human emotion and misguided imagery. It is taught in Chinese philosophy that *shen* naturally rules our lives, but if we lose our balance (which we all do), then the ego and the emotions vie for dominance and *shen* withdraws and becomes hidden. We develop addictions to particular egoistic attitudes and to the emotions that help manifest our egoistic goals. Anger, greed, fear, worry, sorrow, frustration, the perpetual seeking of pleasure in the things of this world of relativity and illusion, are all examples of the types of emotional states that force *shen* into hiding, often for the duration of one's life. But if there is one truth, it is that he or she who seeks *shen* shall find it. As the great Daoist sage Lao Zi said:

> You ask where is Dao?
> Look, it is within your heart!

The great spiritual teachings have all attempted to teach their followers how to temper their excessive desires and unbalanced emotions so that *shen* can naturally regain its position as the ruler of our lives. *Shen* manifests only when the heart is open. Once the heart is open, *shen* manifests as light that illuminates the path of a man or woman in life's journey toward the spiritual goal and along the spiritual path. All people possess *shen*. For some, *shen* manifests easily and early in life. Others must dig for it. In digging for *shen,* one may have to uncover a few or many ugly or unpleasant experiences and thoughts. These thoughts, experiences, and misconceptions provide a kind of cocoon for *shen*. According to Daoist tradition, the great *shen* tonic herbs can help us to find our way into the heart of our own being. They soften the shell and dissolve the barrier. They are a gift from the heart of God.

The *shen* tonics, supported so profoundly by the *jing* and *qi* tonics, have helped me. I have seen them help others as they have helped me, and I know that if you get to know them and make them a part of your life, they will contribute to your life in innumerable, indescribable ways. They are a key to radiant health.

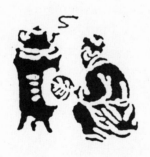

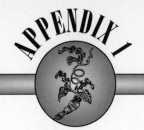

APPENDIX 1

Principal Chinese Herbs and Their Uses

Common Name	Pharmaceutical Name	Botanical or Zoological Name	Pinyin	Chinese	Part Used	Primary Functions
Acanthopanax, Eleutherococcos and Siberian Ginseng	Radix Acanthopanacis	*Acanthopanax senticosus* (Rpr. et Maxim) Harms (China) or *Eleutherococcus senticosus* (Russia)	Ci Wu Ja	刺五加	Root	Adaptogenic. To reinforce *qi*, to invigorate the function of the Spleen and Kidney and to calm the nerves
Achyranthes Root	Radix Achyranthis	*Achyranthes bidentata* B.	Niu Xi	牛膝	Root	Strengthens the bones, joints and ligaments and tonifies the Kidneys and Liver. Invigorates the blood, benefits the lower back and moves energy downward
Aged Citrus Peel, Aged Tangerine Peel	Pericarpium Citri Reticulatae	*Citrus reticulata* Blanco (Rutacaea)	Chen Pi	陈皮	The peel of the ripe tangerines, sun-dried and aged naturally	Regulates *qi* and normalizes the functions of the Spleen and stomach
Albizzia Bark	Cortex Albizzia	*Albizzia julibrisin* Durazz.	He Huan Pi	合欢皮	Bark	To pacify the spirit, calm the mind, and relieve depression
Albizzia Flower	Flos Albizzia	*Albizzia julibrisin* Durazz.	He Huan Hua	合欢花	Flower	Stabilizes *shen*
Alisma	Rhizoma Alismatis	*Alisma orientalis* (Sam.) Juzep. (Alsimataceae)	Ze Xie	泽泻	Tuber	Expelling dampness, inducing urination, and eliminating pathogenic heat by treating false fire conditions of the Kidneys

English Name	Pharmaceutical Name	Botanical Name	Pinyin	Chinese	Part Used	Functions
Amber	Succinum	*Succinum*	Hu Po	琥珀	Fossil resin of Pinaceae, Pinus, which has been buried under ground for thousands of years	To stabilize *shen*
American Ginseng Root	Radix Panacis Quinquefolium	*Panax quinquefolium* L.	Xi Yang Shen	西洋参	Root	An adaptogen, to replenish *qi*, to promote body fluids, to nourish *yin* and clear heat
Asparagus Root	Asparagi Radix/Tuber	*Asparagus cochinchinensis* (Lour.)	Tian Men Dong	天门冬	Tuber	Nourish *yin* and clear heat. Moisten the Lungs and nourish the Kidneys
Astragalus Root	Radix Astragalus	*Astragalus membranaceous* Bge. or *A. mongholicus* Bge	Huang Qi	黄芪	Root	Tonify *qi*, regulate immune functions, strengthen resistance, build blood, strengthen "upright *qi*"
Biota Seed	Semen Biotae Orientalis	*Biota orientalis* (l.) Endl. (Cupressaceae)	Bai Zi Ren	柏子仁	Seed	Nourish the Heart to develop *shen*, tranquilizing to the mind
Bupleurum Root	Radix Bupleuri	*Bupleurum chinese* DC (Umbelliferae)	Chai Hu	柴胡	Root	Harmonizing. Relieves Liver tension and discharges surface heat.
Chrysanthemum Flower	Flos Chrysanthemi	*Chrysanthemum morifolium* Ramat.	Ju hua	菊花	Flower	Clears the Liver and eyes, nourishes *yin* of Kidney and Liver. Disperses heat and wind.

Common Name	Pharmaceutical Name	Botanical or Zoological Name	Pinyin	Chinese	Part Used	Primary Functions
Cinnamon Bark	Cortex Cinnamomi Cassiae	*Cinnamomum cassia* Presl. (Lauraceae)	Rou Gui	肉桂	Inner bark of the trunk and thick branches, from which the outer cork has been scraped off	Supplementing fire of the vital gate to strengthen *yang*, dispelling cold to relieve pain, warming up and clearing the channels
Cinnamon Twig	Ramulus Cinnamomi Cassiae	*Cinnamomum cassia* Blume	Gui Zhi	桂枝	Twig	Promotes the circulation of *qi* and blood. Unblocks *yang* and disperses cold.
Cistanches	Herba Cistanches	*Cistanche deserticola* Y.C. (Orobanchaceae)	Rou Cong Rong	肉苁蓉	Pulpy stem	Tonifying the Kidneys, reinforcing *yang*, replenishing vital Essence and blood, moistening the bowels
Cnidium Seed	Semen Cnidii	*Cnidium Monnieri* (L.) Cusson	She Chuang Zi	蛇床子	Seeds	Tonifies *yang*, warms the Kidneys
Codonopsis Root	Codonopsis Pilosulae, Radix	*Codonopsis pilosula* (Franch.) Nannf. (Campanulaceae)	Dang Shen	党参	Root	*Qi* and blood tonic. Tonifies Spleen and Lungs and mildly invigorates *yang*.
Coix	Semen Coix	*Coicis Lacryma-jobi* (Graminaceae)	Yi Yi Ren	薏苡仁	Seeds	Tonic to Spleen and skin, promoting the flow of moisture

Cordyceps, Chinese Caterpillar Fungus, Winterworm	Cordyceps	Cordyceps sinensis (Berk.) (Fungi)	Dong Chong Xia Cao	冬虫夏草		To nourish jing (both yin and yang), to strengthen the Kidneys and Lungs and to tonify qi. To relieve depression of Liver qi.
Cornus	Fructus Corni Officinalis	Cornus officinalis Sieb. et Zucc.	Shan Yu Rou	山萸肉	Fruit	To stabilize the Kidneys and to contain jing. Astringent, preventing or arresting excessive loss of body fluid. Nourishing the Kidneys and Liver.
Crataegus, Hawthorn Fruit or Berry	Fructus Crataegi	Crataegus cuneata Sieb., and Crataegus pinnatifida Bge. var. major N.E. Br. (Rosaceae)	Shan Zha	山楂	Fruit	Relieves food stagnation, reduces excessive cholesterol, and benefits the cardiovascular system
Cuscuta Seed	Semen Cuscuta	Cuscuta chinensis Lam.	Tu Si Zi	菟丝子	Seed	To tonify the Kidneys, benefit yin and yang jing. Astringent.
Dang Gui, Tang Kuei, Dong Quai, Tang Kwei, Chinese Angelica Root	Radix Angelica	Angelica sinensis (Oliv.) Diels (Umbelliferae)	Dang Gui	当归	Root	Blood tonic, blood stimulant, menstruation-corrective, analgesic
Deer Antler	Cornu Cervi Pantotrichum	Cervus Nippon Temminck (Sika Deer), Cervus Elaphus Linnaeus (Cervidae), and others	Lu Rong	鹿茸	Segments of young deer antler	To tonify the Kidneys and Heart, fortify yang, nourish yin, brighten the mind, and lengthen life

359

Common Name	Pharmaceutical Name	Botanical or Zoological Name	Pinyin	Chinese	Part Used	Primary Functions
Dendrobium	Herba Dendrobii	*Dendrobium nobile* Lindl., *D. loddigesii* Rolfe, *D. chrysanthum* Wall., *D. candidum* Wall. ex Lindl., and *D. fimriatum* Hook. var. oculatum Hook. (Orchidaceae)	Shi Hu	石 斛	Stems and leaves	Replenish *yin jing*, generate fluids, and clear heat
Dioscorea, Wild Chinese Yam, Mountain Medicine	Radix Dioscoreae Opositae	*Dioscorea opposita* Thunb.	Shan Yao	山 药	Peeled rhizome	*Qi* tonic, *yin jing* tonic, tonic to *yin* of Lungs and Stomach, astringent to Kidneys
Donkey Skin Glue	Colla Corii Asini	*Equus asinnus* L.	E Jiao	阿 胶	Skin	To nourish the blood, to stop bleeding, to replenish *yin*, and to moisten the lungs
Dragon Bone	Os Draconis	*Os Draconis Fossilia*	Long Gu	龙 骨	Fossilized bones of prehistoric animals such as mastodon, hairy rhinoceros, hipparion, deer, and oxen	Calm and stabilize *shen*, astringent

Common Name	Pharmaceutical	Botanical Source	Pinyin	Chinese	Part Used	Functions
Dried Ginger	Rhizoma Zingiberis	Zingiber officinale Rosc.	Gan jiang	干姜	Rhizome	Warms the body and expels cold
Epimedium, Goat Sex Herb, and the Herb for the Man Who Likes Sex Too Much, Like a Goat	Herba Epimedii	*Epimedium sagittatum* (Sieb. et Zucc.) Maxim., or *E. brevicornum* Maxim., or *E. pubescens* Maxim., or *E. koreanum* Nakai	Yin Yang Huo	淫羊藿	Leaf	To tonify the Kidneys, strengthen *yang*, eliminate dampness, dispel wind, and fortify the defenses
Eucommia Bark	Cortex Eucommiae	*Eucommia ulmoides* Oliv. (Eucommiaceae)	Du Zhong	杜仲	Bark from the trunk of the tree, after having the outer cork scraped off	Nourishing the Kidneys and Liver; strengthening the bones, ligaments, and muscles; hypotensive; and benefiting the uterus and fetus during pregnancy
Ganoderma, Reishi, Reishi mushroom, Ling Zhi	Ganoderma	*Ganoderma lucidum* (Leyss. ex Fr.) Karst. (Polyporaceae)	Ling Zhi	灵芝	Fruiting body, spores, and sometimes the mycelium	Nourishing tonic, tonic to the three treasures (*jing, qi,* and *shen*), builds body resistance, detoxifying, aphrodisiac, sedative, prolongs life and enhances intelligence and wisdom
Gastrodia	Rhizoma Gastrodiae	*Gastrodia elata* Blume	Tian Ma	天麻	Rhizome	Calms the Liver, calms the nerves, controls spasms and tremors, relieves pain
Gecko, Gejie	Gecko	*Gekko gecko* L.	Gejie	蛤蚧	The spine and tail, and usually the flesh of the back	Tonifies *yang* of the Kidney, replenishes *yin* essence of the Kidneys, nourishes *yin* of the Lungs, enhances breathing and internal respiration, and builds blood

Common Name	Pharmaceutical Name	Botanical or Zoological Name	Pinyin	Chinese	Part Used	Primary Functions
Ginkgo biloba	Folium Ginkgo	*Ginkgo biloba*	Yin Xing Ye	银杏叶	Leaf	To promote longevity, antioxidant, free-radical scavenger, improve circulation and memory
Ginseng	Radix Ginseng	*Panax Ginseng* C. A. Meyer	Ren Shen	人参	Root	Tonify *qi*, adaptogenic, immune modulator, prolong life, overcome fatigue, increase blood volume, aid in recovery from illness or trauma, sharpen and calm the mind, stabilize the emotions, counteract stress, and enhance wisdom
Glehnia	Radix Glehniae	*Glehnia littoralis* F. Schmidt ex Miq.	Bei Sha Shen	北沙参	Root	Tonify *yin* and produce fluids. Tonify the Lungs.
Gynostemma	Herba Gynostemma	*Gynostemma pentaphyllum* (Thunb.) Makino	Jiao Gu Lan	绞股篮	Leaf and stems	Adaptogenic, antioxidant, immune modulating, anti-inflammatory, anti-ulcer, respiratory tonic, platelet regulator, anti-hyperlipidemic, cholesterol regulator, anti-obesity, liver protecting, triglyceride lowering, cardiovascular protectant, anti-thrombic, anti-aging agent
Jujube Date, Red Date	Fructus Jujube	*Ziziphus jujuba* Mill.	Da Zao	大枣	Fruit	Replenishes *qi* in the middle burning space (Spleen and stomach), nourishes blood, soothes the mind, moderates the actions of other herbs in a formula

362

Common Name	Pharmaceutical Name	Botanical Name	Pinyin	Chinese	Part	Functions
Licorice Root, Glycyrrhiza	Radix Glycyrrhiza	*Glycyrrhiza uralensis* Fisch. (Leguminosae)	Gan Cao	甘草	Root	Regulates the function of the stomach, invigorates the Spleen, *qi* tonifying, Lung clearing, latent-heat clearing, detoxicant, anti-inflammatory, harmonizing and regulating to the twelve organs
Ligusticum, Cnidium (not to be confused with Cnidium Seed)	Rhizoma Ligustici	*Ligusticum wallichii*	Chuan Xiong	川芎	Rhizome	Vitalizes the blood, promotes the circulation of blood and *qi*, nourishes blood, relieves wind conditions, analgesic
Ligustrum	Fructus Ligustri lucidi	*Ligustrum lucidum* Ait.	Nu Zhen Zi	女贞子	Seed	Tonifies Kidney and Liver *yin*, enhances immune functions, clears heat, brightens the eyes
Lily Bulb	Bulbus Lilii	*Lilium brownii* var. *viridulum* Baker	Bai He	百合	Bulb	Moistens the Lungs, relieves cough, clears heat in the Heart, calms the Mind and stabilizes the Spirit
Lohanguo	Fructus Momordica	*Momordica grosvenori* Swingle	Luo Han Guo	罗汉果	Fruit	Nourishes *yin*, moistens the Lungs, skin, and stomach
Longan	Arillus Longan	*Euphoria longan* (Lour.) steud.	Long Yan Rou	龙眼肉	Aril	Nourishes the blood, calms the mind, strengthens the Spleen, and tonifies *qi*
Lycium Fruit	Fructus Lycii	*Lycium barbarum* L.	Gou Qi Zi	枸杞子	Fruit	Tonifies the Kidneys and promotes the production of essence, strengthens the legs, nourishes the Liver and brightens the eyes, moistens the Lungs

Common Name	Pharmaceutical Name	Botanical or Zoological Name	Pinyin	Chinese	Part Used	Primary Functions
Ma Huang, Ephedra	Herba Ephedrae	*Ephedra sinica* Stapf, or *E. intermedia* Schrenk et Mey, or *E. equisetina* Bge. (Ephedraceae)	Ma Huang	麻黄	Herbaceous stems	Decongestant, diaphoretic, cardiorespiratory stimulant, diuretic, thermogenic and surface relieving
Male Silk Moth	Bombyx mori	*Bombyx mori*	Xiong Can E	雄蚕蛾	Torso	To tonify Kidneys, strengthen male reproductive system, and as an aphrodisiac
Morinda	Radix Morindae	*Morinda officinalis*	Ba Ji Tian	巴戟天	Root	Tonify *yang*, supplement *qi*
Ophiopogon Root	Radix Ophiopononis	*Ophiopogon japonicus* Thunb. Ker-Gawl.; also *Liriope spicata*	Mai Men Dong	麦门冬	Tuberous root	Provide cooling *yin* to the Heart, Lungs, and stomach, to promote production of body fluids, to clear heat in the Heart and relieve irritability, to relieve dry cough, dry mouth and tongue, and to moisten the bowels
Pearl	Margarita	*Pteria margaitifera* (L.) or *P. martensil* (Dunker)	Zhen Zhu	珍珠	Whole pearl	*Shen* stabilizing, generate beautiful skin and clear toxins
Placenta	Placenta hominis or Placenta bovis	*P. hominis* or *P. bovis*	Zi He Che	紫河车	Cleaned, boiled placenta	Tonifies *yang* and nourishes *yin jing*, builds *qi* and blood

Polygala Root, Will Strengthener	Radix Polygalae	*Polygala tenuifolia* Willd.	Yuan Zhi	远 志	Root	To calm the Heart and mind, to clear the orifices, to resolve phlegm and to strengthen the will
Polygonatum, Solomonseal Root	Rhizome Polygonati	*Polygonatum sibircum*	Huang Jing	黄 精	Root	To nourish the *qi* of the Heart, to strengthen the mind, to nourish the marrow, to moisten the Lungs
Polygonum Stem	Caulis Polygoni Multiflori	*Polygonum multiflorum* Thunb.	Ye Jiao Teng	夜 交 藤	Stem	Nourish Heart blood, steady the mind, stabilize *shen*, promote sound sleep
Polygonum, Shou Wu, and sometimes erroneously Fo Ti	Radix Polygonum	*Polygonum multiflorum* Thunb. (Polygonaceae)	He Shou Wu	何 首 乌	Tuberous root	As a tonic to the Kidney and Liver functions, toning up the vital Essence and blood, fortifying the muscles, tendons, and bones, and to prevent premature aging, maintaining the youthful condition and color of the hair, strengthening sperm and ova, fortifying the back and knees, and as the premier longevity herb of Chinese tonic herbalism
Polyporus	Polyporus	*Polyporus umbellata* (pers) Fr.	Zhu Ling	猪 苓	Fungal mass	Dispersing moisture, promoting water metabolism, improving immune functions

Common Name	Pharmaceutical Name	Botanical or Zoological Name	Pinyin	Chinese	Part Used	Primary Functions
Polyrachis, or Ant	Polyrachis	*Polyrhachis vicina* Roger	Ma Yi	螞蟻	Whole dried ants	Promotes, maintains, and prolongs life, replenishes *qi*, nourishes blood, increases vitality, adaptogenic, regulates *yin* and *yang*, antiaging, enhances immunocompetence (bipolar immune regulation), improves sexual function and increases virility and fertility, strengthens musculoskeletal system, calms anxiety, promotes sound sleep, improves digestion and assimilation
Poria, Hoelen (note: the name Hoelen is not used in China but has recently taken hold in America)	Poria	*Poria cocos* (Schw.) wolf	Fu Ling	茯苓	Fungal mass	To strengthen the Spleen and transform dampness, to stabilize *shen* and calm the mind
Prepared Aconite	Radix Aconiti Lateralis Praeparata	*Aconitum carmichaeli* Debs.	Fu Zi	附子	Lateral roots, specially prepared	To supplement fire of the vital gate to strengthen *yang*. Aconite warms the interior of the body and dispels cold.
Prepared Rehmannia	Radix Rehmanniae praparatae	*Rehmannia glutinosa* Libosch.	Shu Di Huang	熟地黃	Tuberous root	To tonify the Kidneys and nourish *yin jing*

Common Name	Pharmaceutical	Botanical	Pinyin	Chinese	Part Used	Properties
Prince Ginseng	Radix Pseudostellariae	*Pseudostellaria hererophylla* (Miq.) Pax ex Pax et Hoffm.	Tai Zi Shen	太子参	Tuberous root	Builds *qi* and generates body fluids
Notoginseng, San Qi, Tian Qi or Pseudoginseng	Radix Notoginseng or Radix Pseudoginseng	*Panax notoginseng* (Burk) Chen	San Qi or Tian Qi	三七	Root	Cooked: as a blood and *yin* tonic; raw: to stop bleeding and transform congealed blood
Pueraria Root	Radix Puerariae	*Pueraria lobata* (Willd.) Ohwi.	Ge Gen	葛根	Root	Releases tension, heat and congestion in the muscles, especially of the upper back. Nourishes fluids.
Royal Jelly	Secretio Apis Mellifera	*Apis mellifera*	Feng Wang Jiang	蜂王浆	Secretion	Nourishes blood, *yin* and *qi*
Salvia Root	Radix Salvia Miltiorrhizae	*Salvia miltiorrhiza* Bge.	Dan Shen	丹参	Root	Invigorates the blood and reduces blood stagnation. Clears heat and reduces irritability.
Schizandra, Five Flavor Fruit	Fructus Schizandra	*Schizandra chinensis*	Wu Wei Zi	五味子	Fruit with seed	Broad spectrum adaptogenic, promotes beauty, tonifies Kidneys, rejuvenates the Lungs, purifies Liver, eliminates toxins, astringent, tonifies all three treasures
Sea Dragon	Sygnathus	*Sygnathoides biaculeatus*	Hai Long	海龙	Whole dried fish	*Yang* tonic, sexual tonic
Sea Horse	Hippocampus	*Hippocampus*	Hai Ma	海马	Whole dried fish	Provides *yang* to the Kidneys, aphrodisiac

Common Name	Pharmaceutical Name	Botanical or Zoological Name	Pinyin	Chinese	Part Used	Primary Functions
Spirit Poria	Spirit Poria	*Poria cocos* (Schw.) wolf and *Pinus longa*	Fu Ling	茯 苓	Whole fungus with hostwood	To stabilize *shen* and calm the mind, to strengthen the Spleen and transform dampness
Tortoise Shell	Plastrum Testudinis	*Chenemus reevesii* (Gray)	Gui Ban	龟 板	Pastron (undershell) of a freshwater tortoise	To nourish *yin* and subdue fire (hyperactive *yang*), to tonify the Kidneys and to strengthen the skeleton, and to cause the *qi* to ascend
Turtle Shell	Carapx Trionycis	*Trionyx sinensis* Wiegmann	Bie Jia	鳖 甲	Shell of freshwater turtle	To nourish *yin* and subdue fire ("unruly *yang*"), to soften hardness
Walnut Kernel	Semen Juglandis	*Juglans regia* L.	Hu Tao Ren	胡 桃 仁	Kernel (Seed)	To tonify the functions of the Kidneys, strengthen the lower back, relieve cough due to Lung deficiency, relieve constipation due to dryness, and to benefit the skin
White Atractylodes	Rhizoma Atractylodis Macrocephalae	*Atractylodes macrocephala* Koidz.	Bai Zhu	白 术	Rhizome	*Qi* tonic, aids digestion and invigorates the *yang*.
White Peony Root	Radix Paeoniae alba	*Paeonia lactiflora* pall.	Bai Shao	白 芍	Root	To nourish blood and consolidate *yin*, to soothe the Liver, to cleanse the blood, and to stop pain
Zizyphus Seed	Semen Zizyphi spinosae	*Zizyphus spinosa* Hu	Suan Zao Ren	酸 枣 仁	Seed	Nourishes Heart blood, pacifies *shen*, benefits *yin*

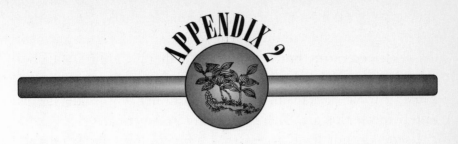

Sources of Chinese Herbal Products

Quality Chinese herbs are readily available at Chinese herb shops located in predominantly Asian districts of many cities in America. You may be able to obtain raw herbs such as Ginseng, Astralagus, Dan Gui, Schizandra, and most of the other herbs described in this book at these herb shops; a few herbs—such as Gynostemma, Duanwood Reishi, Tibetan Cordyceps, and Acanthopanax root (Siberian Ginseng)—are more difficult to find. As emphasized throughout the book, most herbs come in a variety of qualities and grades. Try to avoid the lower-quality grades, as superior-grade herbs will likely yield much better results. Solicit the advice of the staff at these herb shops and always ask to see the highest grades.

Most natural food stores now feature a wide range of herbal products. Most, however, do not sell bulk herbs. The products sold in natural foods stores range in quality. This book can help you make educated decisions. Do not rely on standardization as the sole basis of decision making. Read the labels carefully and read each company's product literature. Avoid low-end brands. But remember that the content, not fancy labels, make a product potent.

Professional herbalists are another excellent source of tonic herbal products. These herbalists may be pure herbalists, or they may be Gung Fu teachers, Qi Gung teachers, acupuncturists, knowledgeable multilevel marketers, or even physicians. As described in the body of the book, there is a difference between *medical* herbalism and *tonic* herbalism. If you are interested in tonic herbalism, find a practitioner who understands and respects this art. There are many in America.

If you do not have access to a Chinese herb shop, reliable mail-order sources are listed below.

Ron Teeguarden's Herbarium

Supplier of bulk herbs and tonics, including a collection of rare tonic herbs. Offers over 200 formulations, both classical and specially designed. Call or E-mail for a detailed catalogue, additional literature, information on private consultations by appointment, details about the Radiant Health News newsletter or Web site, and referrals to tonic herbal practitioners in your area.

P.O. Box 42030
Los Angeles, CA 90049
Phone: 310-471-0404
Fax: 310-471-9174
E-mail: rons_herbarium@hotmail.com
       radiant_health@hotmail.com

Brion Herbs Corporation

The manufacturer of the Sun Ten brand of herbal products, Brion is a supplier of ready-made, spray-dried Chinese herbal powders, capsules, and pills, including over 400 classical formulas and a number of newly developed products. Their products are sold primarily through practitioners; contact the company for someone in your area who carries them.

9200 Jeronimo Rd.
Irvine, CA 92618
Phone: 714-587-1238
Fax: 1-800-557-1260
E-mail: brionc@sunten.com

Wing Hop Fung Ginseng and Herb Company
Suppliers of all the standard Chinese herbs in bulk, the company also carries many patent formulas and tonic preparations. Visit one of their stores, or order by mail:
727 North Broadway Ave.
Los Angeles, CA 90012
Phone: 213-346-9688

Mycoherb
MycoHerb produces superior concentrates derived from nutritive fungi grown organically on whole grain. They produce a number of excellent products featuring Chinese tonic mushrooms. Call for information and for practitioners and other outlets that sell their high-quality products.
P.O. Box 1844
Burlingame, CA 94011
Phone: 650-343-9840
Fax: 650-343-2704

Jen-On Pharmaceutical
Jen-On is a fine Chinese herbal manufacturer selling a nice range of superior tonic formulations and individual herbs in concentrated form. Their quality is quite good. Contact them for shops and practitioners in your area who distribute their products.
1015 S. Nogales St. Suite 120
Rowland Heights, CA 91748
Phone: 818-965-0906
Fax: 818-965-6162

K'an Herb Company
K'an Herb Company provides high-quality Chinese herbal formulas. K'an's formulas are distributed through health professionals. Contact K'an for a list of health practitioners in your area.
6001 Butler Lane
Scotts Valley, CA 95066
Phone: 408-438-9450
Fax: 408-438-9457

Radiant Health Corporation
Radiant Health markets Chinese tonic products via mail order as well as multi-level marketing.
520 Barsana Road
Austin, TX 78737-9075
Phone: 800-274-7325

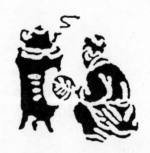

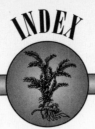

INDEX